Bariatric Surgery Patients

Patients

A NUTRITIONAL GUIDE

Bariatric Surgery Patients
A NUTRITIONAL GUIDE

Betty Wedman-St Louis

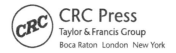

CRC Press
Taylor & Francis Group
Boca Raton London New York

CRC Press is an imprint of the
Taylor & Francis Group, an **informa** business

CRC Press
Taylor & Francis Group
6000 Broken Sound Parkway NW, Suite 300
Boca Raton, FL 33487-2742

© 2017 by Taylor & Francis Group, LLC
CRC Press is an imprint of Taylor & Francis Group, an Informa business

No claim to original U.S. Government works

Printed on acid-free paper
Version Date: 20161104

International Standard Book Number-13: 978-1-4987-6561-9 (Paperback)

Library of Congress Cataloging-in-Publication Data

Names: Wedman-St Louis, Betty, author.
Title: Bariatric surgery patients : a nutritional guide / Betty Wedman-St Louis.
Description: Boca Raton : Taylor & Francis, 2017. | Includes bibliographical references
and index.
Identifiers: LCCN 2016024604| ISBN 9781498765619 (pbk. : alk. paper) | ISBN
9781498765657 (e-book)
Subjects: | MESH: Obesity--diet therapy | Obesity--surgery | Obesity--rehabilitation |
Bariatric Surgery--rehabilitation | Diet, Reducing
Classification: LCC RD540 | NLM WD 210 | DDC 617.4/3--dc23
LC record available at https://lccn.loc.gov/2016024604

Visit the Taylor & Francis Web site at
http://www.taylorandfrancis.com

and the CRC Press Web site at
http://www.crcpress.com

This book is dedicated to Alfredo Fernandez, MD, who educates his patients about the importance of nutrition with more compassion than most physicians

and

to the many bariatric surgery patients who have changed their eating and lifestyle habits to achieve a better quality of life.

Contents

Preface

As a clinical nutritionist, every day I hear about the confusion and frustrations that people experience about nutrition and the food supply. From my undergraduate days at the University of Minnesota until the present, it has been a personal and professional disappointment to watch Big Tobacco become Big Food. Sadly, I have observed government officials being influenced by food industry lobbyists to promote margarine and wine as being healthy.

Over the past 40 years, the recommended diet for weight loss has gone from a chew and count diet (chew small bites and count each mouthful swallowed) to a $30 billion business of diet books, supplements, special meals, and exercise equipment with personal trainers. Nowhere do you hear the "Less Is More" message about food, or that eating home-prepared meals lowers diabetes risk. Instead, costly weight loss programs produce a 5–10 lb. reduction, which lasts about 4 weeks before the pounds are regained.

Bariatric surgery is a feasible and beneficial option for effective weight management, provided multiple modifications are made in a person's lifestyle—food choices, physical activity, stress management, and dietary supplementation—to meet nutritional needs. Surgical weight loss programs need regular visits to health-care professionals to ensure they have a diet and supplement plan for long-term weight loss and improvement in quality of life. Bariatric surgery is a tool—one of many that can assist in obesity management—but lifestyle changes make the difference in permanent weight loss.

Research has yet to discover a "fat" gene in humans to explain the obesity epidemic, but as Johnson and Andrews point out in *Evolutionary Anthropology*, there are "thrifty" genes. Too much food and too little activity is leading to over 200,000 bariatric surgeries annually in the United States costing from $15,000–$30,000 per patient. Each of these surgical candidates needs a personalized nutrition plan, activity regime, and lifestyle alterations to insure weight loss success.

Americans believe obesity is a national health crisis but do not place much blame on junk food or the responsibility on too much time spent on television, computers, or video games *and* the widespread availability of cheap fast food. They spend more time watching food-related television shows than cooking their own food. Many patients proudly tell me they do not know how to cook and could not care less about learning. These patients put more value in what they watch on television or post on the Internet than in what goes into their body.

This bariatric surgery nutrition guide is designed as a practical, easy-to-read and use publication for health-care professionals whose responsibility is to help patients be more accountable for their own health through weight reduction.

Betty Wedman-St Louis, PhD, RD, LD
Clinical Nutritionist
Private Practice
St. Petersburg, Florida
www.betty-wedman-stlouis.com

Introduction

Morbid obesity is a worldwide disease that is associated with a variety of medical conditions, which may shorten life and lead to huge health-care expenses. This disease has become a pandemic since the late twentieth century. The expanding waistline is an unhealthy trend and applies to all ages as a major health problem. The primitive prevention efforts addressing this public health concern have not been able to cope with the problem, and morbid obesity has continued to progress unimpeded.

The World Health Organization (WHO) defines overweight and obesity as an accumulation of fat in excess that presents as a health risk. The basic measurement for evaluating the general population is calculating the body mass index (BMI). This is a person's weight in kilograms or pounds divided by the individual's square of the height in meters or feet. An individual with a BMI equal to or more than 25 is considered overweight and a BMI of 30 is considered obese. Those with a BMI above 40 are morbidly obese and this group suffers the greatest impact on their health. Those who are morbidly obese are at greater risk for illness including diabetes, high blood pressure, sleep apnea, gastroesophageal reflux disease (GERD), gallstones, osteoarthritis, heart disease, and cancer. In 2013, the American Medical Association (AMA) classified obesity as a chronic disease. There were debates in 2013 between committees which said that "medicalizing" obesity would include one-third of all Americans and describe them as being ill. The fear was the potential impact on the reliance for costly drugs and surgery.

Approximately, 65% of our population is overweight and 12% are morbidly obese. This is despite more than 25 years of attempted medical management. Clearly all current efforts have failed to control this enormous problem. Could it be that we have failed to recognize the cause of the disease and therefore have misdirected our efforts?

In the past 50–60 years we have completely changed what we eat. Recent studies indicate that many of the new foods and oils are having a direct impact on central regulatory systems in our body and are thought to be among the main culprits resulting in obesity. Until we disseminate this information, we will not be able to control the problem.

Bariatric surgery is a unique field, in that with one operation, a person can potentially be cured of numerous medical diseases including diabetes, hypertension, high cholesterol, sleep apnea, chronic headaches, venous stasis disease, urinary incontinence, liver disease, and arthritis. It is the only proven method that results in durable weight loss and offers a viable solution for patients who have tried and failed to lose weight though dieting. This proven surgical approach, combined with the marked improvement in quality of life and the quick recovery with minimally invasive techniques, has fueled the surge in the number of bariatric procedures performed annually since the beginning of this century. Yet we are only operating on approximately 1% of those who qualify for surgery.

Bariatric surgery (weight loss surgery) includes a variety of procedures performed on individuals that are diagnosed with the chronic disease of obesity. Weight loss is achieved by reducing the transit time of food from the mouth to the small intestine. This results in major hormonal changes leading to weight loss and major changes in gut bacteria that also enhance weight loss. This protocol must be complemented with a complete lifestyle change avoiding those foods that have been identified as part of the problem. Extended studies show the procedures cause significant long-term loss of weight, recovery from diabetes, and improvement in cardiovascular risk factors. Mortality decreases from 40% to 23%.

The U.S. Institutes of Health recommends bariatric surgery for those individuals with a BMI of at least 40 and for those with a BMI of 35 and serious coexisting medical conditions such as diabetes or cardiovascular disease. Research is emerging that indicates bariatric surgery could be appropriate for those with a BMI of 35–40 with no comorbidities or a BMI of 30–35 with significant comorbidities. The most recent American Society for Metabolic and Bariatric Surgery (ASMBS) guidelines suggest that any patient with a BMI of more than 30 with comorbidities is a candidate for bariatric surgery.

The advent of "open" weight loss surgery started in the 1950s. It involved an intestinal bypass by anastomosing the upper and lower intestine, bypassing a large portion of the absorptive circuit and causing weight loss solely by the malabsorption of food. In 1963, Drs. Howard Payne, Lorent DeWind, and Robert Commons developed the jejunocolic shunt, which connects the upper small intestine to the colon. Two years later, Dr. Edward Mason and Chikashi Ito, physicians at the University of Iowa, developed the original gastric bypass for weight reduction. This procedure has fewer complications than the intestinal bypass and for this reason Dr. Mason is known as the "father of obesity surgery."

No procedure is perfect but the majority of patients have a successful clinical outcome. Patients need to decide through an honest discussion with a bariatric surgeon which procedure may be best suited for them. New techniques and innovations are ongoing and patients and surgeons should embrace change but credit the lessons learned from the pioneers.

Alfredo Fernandez, MD, FASMBS
Bariatric Surgery Medical Director, Brandon Regional Hospital
Bariatric Surgery Medical Director, Florida Hospital—Carrollwood
Bariatric Surgery Medical Director, Tampa Community Hospital
General Surgery Adjunct Professor, Barry University

Author

Dr. Betty Wedman-St Louis is a licensed nutritionist specializing in kidney disease, diabetes, digestive diseases, bariatric surgery nutrition, and cancer who has been in private practice for over 40 years. Her BS in food and nutrition from the University of Minnesota introduced her to how the food industry influences eating habits. Dr. Wedman-St Louis completed her MS in nutrition at Northern Illinois University where she studied the relationship between weightlessness and prolonged bed rest on potassium requirements in adults. She completed a clinical internship at the Mayo Clinic where she began to understand that allopathic medicine did not have answers to many nutrition issues. Dr. Wedman-St Louis practiced at the Hinsdale Medical Center, Hinsdale, Illinois, before completing her PhD in nutrition and environmental health from The Union Institute in Cincinnati. Dr. Wedman-St Louis completed her doctorate internship in multimedia production for distance learning and online course development at WUSF-Tampa. She is the author of numerous published articles on current nutrition topics including phosphates in foods, folate, Vitamin B_{12}, seafood nutrition, alpha lipoic acid, and diabetes. She has also authored columns for the *Hinsdale Doings*, *Chicago Sun Times*, *Columbia Missourian*, and the *Tampa Bay Times* and has taught undergraduate and graduate courses on nutrition and related topics.

1

SELLING OBESITY—FOOD AS A CHEAP AND LEGAL DRUG

Today, a growing majority of people have changed their food choices according to illogical and misdirected concepts from the food industry, which has resulted in wasted food and money and a threat to public health. Each pound of body fat represents wasted food whether it is on the waistline or in the landfill. All the while, the food industry has enjoyed watching Americans gain weight while they reaped the financial rewards.

During the past 60 years, the U.S. food industry has been remarkably successful in merging small family farms into giant corporations while families that previously cooked at home now buy and consume almost half their meals prepared outside the home. The food service sector of the U.S. economy generates trillions of dollars in sales annually and accounts for 13% of the U.S. gross national product (GNP) while employing 17% of the nation's labor force [1, p. 11]. Marion Nestle, professor of nutrition at New York University, points out in *Food Politics* that the public spends $800 billion annually on food and drink with $90 billion going to alcoholic beverages [1, p. 11].

Economic pressures in agriculture, poor government policies, and the food industry sponsorship of nutrition professionals, their continuing education programs, and publications have produced the obesity crisis. Dr. Nestle outlines how food companies influence government nutrition policy through lobbyists and political action committee contributions to candidates [1, p. 12]. She also describes how health-care professionals, including dietitians, are influenced by corporate-sponsored education and research activities through consulting payments, lectures, memberships on advisory boards, and sponsorships of professional journals.

The very nutritional professionals who were supposed to teach and guide the policy makers to make better public health policy in order to help avert the obesity crisis were won over by the food industry. At a recent American Dietetic Association's Annual Meeting—now the Academy of Nutrition and Dietetics—more than 30 food, beverage, and nutrition supplement companies provided sessions with sponsored speakers who offered attendees free gifts and/or coupons for patients. No wonder it is hard to determine what is healthy when nutrition professionals are industry promoters instead of creative thinkers.

Joseph Mercola, doctor of osteopathic medicine (DO), illustrated the food industry ties to the most widely known academic institution in the field of nutrition—the American Society for Nutrition (ASN). Three academic journals including the *American Journal of Clinical Nutrition* are published by the organization. In June 2015, Michele Simon, a public health law attorney for 20 years, was interviewed by Dr. Mercola in his online newsletter. She stated, "Food, beverage, supplement, biotech, and pharmaceutical industry leaders are able to purchase cozy relationships with the nation's top nutrition researchers" [2] and revealed the disturbing ties between the ASN and the primary purveyors of obesity and chronic diseases [3].

The obesity crisis has been caused by three significant changes in our food and nutrition policy during the past 50 years. Each one of these factors needs to be modified individually and nationally if the obesity battle is to be won.

High-fat and **high-sugar foods** need to be replaced with unprocessed real foods that do not contain additives and preservatives, artificial colors, and flavors.

Alcohol consumption provides empty calories that may increase the government taxation bottom line but only causes inflammation in the brain and liver.

Sedentary lifestyles need to be modified and Americans educated to put away their electronics long enough each day to increase oxygen uptake and muscle movement for improved nutrient and waste recycling in every cell of the body.

Food is necessary to human survival yet many people have problems controlling the quantity and quality. Obesity extracts a tremendous cost in the form of disease risk and physical encumbrance. The addictive properties of food can trigger compulsive eating behaviors in a drug-like manner [4, p. 39].

Neurobiological effects of sugar and simple carbohydrates described by Haddock and Dill in *Food as a Drug* lead to habitual and difficult to control reactions similar to drug addiction. The addict becomes dependent on the mood or behavior effects of the drug or sugar [4, p. 20]. One explanation is that high-carbohydrate meals alter tryptophan levels that stimulate 5-hydroxytryptophan (5-HTP) synthesis. The elevation of 5-HTP level leads to carbohydrate ingestion. When protein is consumed, the tryptophan and 5-HTP decrease, and the individual craves carbohydrates again, leading to the overeating cycle [4, p. 39].

Questions about whether sugar and high-glycemic carbohydrates can act as potent psychoactive drugs in the obesity model abound. Convincing obese individuals that they are powerless to control their intake of sugar and high-glycemic carbohydrates may lead to feelings of deprivation and low self-esteem, but that only increases the parallel between foods and drugs. Sweet cravings were associated with opiate addiction by Willenbring et al. in 1989. The opiate antagonist naloxone has been shown to be helpful in reducing sweet and high-fat snack preferences [4, p. 130].

Schulte et al. propose that highly processed foods share pharmacokinetic properties—such as concentrated dose and rapid rate of absorption—with abused drugs. The fat and high-glycemic carbohydrates are rapidly absorbed into the blood creating an addiction-like eating behavior [5]. Professor Sidney Mintz sheds light on how sugar became such an addictive substance in *Sweetness and Power: The Place of Sugar in Modern History*. As a food anthropologist he writes

> In 1000 AD, few Europeans knew of the existence of sucrose, or cane sugar. But soon afterward they learned about it; by 1650 in England the nobility and the wealthy had become inveterate sugar eaters, and sugar figured in their medicine, literary imagery, and displays of rank. By no later than 1800 sugar had become necessity in the diet of every English person; by 1900, it was supplying nearly one-fifth of the calories in the English diet ... That human beings like the taste of sweetness does not explain why some eat immense quantities of sweet foods and others hardly any [6].

The thesis of Dr. Mintz's work was to identify that food choices are related to availability and that preferences are identified at the center of an individual's self-definition. Food advertisements—especially those of the high-sugar soda producers—focus on the self-identity issue.

Winning the battle against high-fat and high-sugar foods is not an easy task when food companies like Coca Cola, the world's largest producer of sugary beverages, fund studies stating that the new "science-based" solution to the obesity crisis is to maintain a healthy weight by getting more exercise and not worrying about calories [7]. The company backed a nonprofit organization of professors at three U.S. universities called the Global Energy Balance Network whose message was meant to divert criticism away from the role sugary drinks have played in the obesity crisis.

In *Soda Politics*, Marion Nestle described the research organization as a "front group for Coca Cola's agenda to confuse the science and deflect attention from dietary intake" [7].

Coca Cola and the other carbonated beverages contain 10 teaspoons of sugar in a 12 oz. can. That is more sugar in one can of soda than what the World Health Organization (WHO) recommends in an entire day. (WHO recommends no more than 6 teaspoons of sugar per day.) The high amount of fructose corn syrup, refined salts, and caffeine found in many sodas can contribute to high blood pressure, diabetes, and obesity.

Food Cravings

Food cravings or the desire to eat a specific food have been studied using functional magnetic resonance imaging (fMRI) to explore the neurological basis of cravings. The imaging data suggests that areas of the amygdala, anterior cingulate, orbital frontal cortex, insula, hippocampus, caudate, and dorsolateral prefrontal cortex are activated during periods when yearning for a food [8].

Clemens and Smit explain the desire for chocolate consumption because of its mood-altering endogenous compounds—phenylethylamine, tyramine, serotonin, tryptophan, and magnesium. Cravings may result from a sense of deprivation or reaction to stress [9].

Food cravings do not represent a nutrient deficiency but result in abnormal behaviors of psychosocial nature caused by socio-cultural factors, stressful environments, or hormonal fluctuations [10]. Thus, the food industry capitalizes on its benefit through food cues that influence the desire to eat even after finishing a meal. Food cues come in many forms from emotions in television advertising, images in print, or other media to aromas at the supermarket. As Americans watch more food shows on television, they eat more processed foods at restaurants and at home.

"American consumers have permanently changed their eating habits. The era of three square meals a day has gone the way of the typewriter and vacuum tube," research firm Packaged Facts, Rockville, Maryland, notes in a recent report [11]. Nutrition bars and granola bars are replacing traditional meals to the tune of $5.5 billion reported in November 2014. Mintel, a Chicago-based research firm that studies food trends has attributed this increase in bar sales to the obesity epidemic and a desire for healthier choices. Dessert bars allow guilt-free indulgence and a small treat that is perceived healthier than a candy bar. "You deserve it all—health, happiness, and daily indulgences," says Skinnygirl Daily on its website [11].

Most nutrition and granola bars are super sweet with high sugar content and little to no advantage over a traditional candy bar. To win more health conscious consumers, the food industry is beginning to use alternatives to refined sugar. Brown rice syrup, date syrup, and coconut sugar are still high glycemic and contain the same simple carbohydrates and calorie count.

Fast Foods = Cheap and Legal Drug Effect

McDonalds and other fast-food companies have mastered the art of product appeal through availability, price, chemical composition, and marketing [12]. So whether feeding a family or a hunger, cheap food is very addictive. The quick dopamine response from eating causes an instant feeling of satiation and pleasure that reinforces a repeat performance the next time hunger strikes. Lawsuits filed by consumers against fast-food companies have largely been ignored by the media despite public health issues cited in the suits [13].

American schools are profiting from the sale of fast food through the National School Lunch Program. Established in 1946 by President Harry Truman, the program was designed to provide nutritionally balanced, low-cost, or free lunches to children each school day.

Instead, the meals served today consist of high calories, refined sugar, and fatty choices fueling the obesity crisis [14]. The U.S. government is essentially funding a program that promotes, not prevents, obesity [1, p. 13].

Big Tobacco Becomes Big Food

Food and beverage companies have expanded to enormous size in just the past 25 years. In 2000, seven U.S. companies—Philip Morris, ConAgra, Mars, IBP, Sara Lee, Heinz, and Tyson Foods—ranked among the 10 largest food companies in the world. Nestle (Switzerland) ranked first and Unilever (U.K./Netherlands) third with Danone (France) sixth. By 1997 just three U.S. companies—Philip Morris (+ Kraft Foods + Miller Brewing), ConAgra, and RJR-Nabisco—accounted for ~20% of all food expenditures [1, p. 13]. Mergers among food and cigarette companies—R.J. Reynolds and Philip Morris particularly—led to unprecedented control of the processed food industry. A few of the food industry mergers are as follows [1, p. 13]:

Nestle: Carnation foods, Lean Cuisine, Butterfinger Candy

Unilever: Lipton tea, Wishbone salad dressing, Best Foods, Thomas English muffins, Skippy peanut butter, Ben & Jerry's ice cream, Slim Fast

Philip Morris: Kraft Foods, Jello, Altoid Mints

Pepsico: Pepsi, Diet Pepsi, Lay's potato chips, Tropicana fruit juices

Kellogg: Cereals, Eggo frozen waffles

Eat More–Eat More

In the competitive food arena, each company must satisfy stockholders by gaining increasing market share through expanding sales by advertising and developing "new" products. In recent years, the portion size of a serving has increased to encourage greater sales while feeding the obesity epidemic. Portion distortion surrounds today's supermarket shoppers. They may not realize how dinner plates, cereal bowls, and glasses have changed to accommodate larger portions since the end of the twentieth century.

New product introductions in the 1980s were fewer than 6,000 annually but by 1995, the food industry had introduced 16,900 new food and beverage products [1, p. 13]. Fortunately, the size of supermarkets allows *only* 50,000–65,000 items from the current estimate of over 320,000 items competing for shelf space [15].

Portion Distortion

Portion distortion can be seen in how the size of bagels has changed over the past 20 years. A bagel 20 years ago was 3 inches in diameter and had 140 kcal. Today a bagel is 5–6 inches in diameter and has 350 kcal.

Pizza serving sizes 20 years ago were two medium wedges totaling 500 kcal. Today a pizza serving is 2 large wedges providing 850 kcal.

French fry servings have greatly changed during the same 20-year period. In the 1980s and 1990s a 2.4 oz. serving had 222 kcal. Today the serving size is 5.4 oz. with 500 kcal.

Plate and glass sizes also influence serving sizes. A 1960s dinner plate was no more than 8–9 inches, but today the average dinner plate is 12 inches. Each extra inch of dinner plate can add 200–400 extra kcal to a meal.

Many techniques have been suggested to help individuals learn to eat less and better judge what a health portion is. Everything from a tennis ball = 1 cup rice or pasta or ice cream to a golf ball as a serving size for peanut butter has been proposed, but since there is no standard serving size for foods commonly eaten, no authoritative source is available to assist in this learning process. Here are some additional ways to teach appropriate serving sizes:

1 deck of cards = 3 oz. chicken
1 domino = 1 oz. cheese
1 die = 1 teaspoon butter or margarine
1 baseball = medium fruit serving
1 female fist = 1 cup pasta or noodles
1 golf ball = 2 tablespoons salad dressing
1 packet dental floss = 1 oz. chocolate
1 computer mouse = baked potato

Food Frauds

Food frauds abound in the supermarket as consumers are demanding greater "value added" for their purchases while not wanting to pay more. Cheap food leads to expensive health care: obesity surgery to poor animal welfare, and artificial colors and flavors being labeled as *food*.

A 2014 article by Joseph Mercola, titled "Why Won't Walmart's Ice Cream Sandwiches Melt?" is a prime example of how gums and additives create new-to-nature food ingredients that allow ice creams to no longer melt [16].

A look at the ingredients in Walmart's Great Value Vanilla Flavored Ice Cream Sandwiches reads like a chemistry book:

> **Ice Cream** (milk, cream, buttermilk, sugar, whey, corn syrup, contains 1% or less mono-and diglycerides, vanilla extract, guar gum, calcium sulfate, carob bean gum, cellulose gum, carrageenan, artificial flavor, annatto for color)

> **Wafers** (wheat flour, sugar, soybean oil, palm oil, cocoa, dextrose, caramel color, corn syrup, high-fructose corn syrup, corn flour, food starch-modified, salt, soy lecithin, baking soda, artificial flavor)

Another food fraud of which consumers need to be aware is farm-raised seafood, which is reported to be an excellent source of omega-3 fatty acids. Farm-raised catfish, trout, and salmon are fed fish pellets from corn, soy, wheat, and "pelagic species which are not used for human consumption" [17].

According to Dr. Joyce Nettleton in *Seafood Nutrition*, the omega-3 fatty acids in fish are derived from the phytoplankton in the food chain that fish eat [18]. Corn, soy, and wheat do not contain phytoplankton.

Honey tops the list of food frauds because United States consumption is approximately 400 million pounds per year—approximately 1.3 pounds per person according to the U.S. Department of Agriculture (USDA), but the nation's beekeepers can only supply approximately 48% of what is needed. The remaining 52% comes from Asian countries—particularly China—which are notorious for exporting products that are contaminated with antibiotics, heavy metals, or corn syrup [19].

Another food fraud is the remaking of orange juice from concentrate that has color, flavor, and synthetic folic acid that are not safe for consumers because they can mask Vitamin B_{12} deficiency. According to researchers at the Max Planck Institute in Germany, these "remade" juices fortified with folic acid can lose an average of 46% of the nutrient during a year's storage when kept in an environment reflective of supermarket refrigeration. When the juices were exposed to light degradation, the nutrient loss was even worse—especially during the first 6 months of storage [20].

Vitamin water is the epitome of deception and unsubstantiated claims according to the Center for Science in the Public Interest (CSPI). Coca Cola's notion that "you can take a penny's worth of vitamins and minerals and mix them with a sugary drink and convert them to something healthful" is bogus, according to David Schardt, a senior nutritionist at CSPI [21].

Everyone Eats

Since everyone eats, the term "mindful eating" or sustainable food choices is now an approach to change food habits, reduce effectiveness of advertising on food choices, and promote more food preparation instead of grabbing a candy or granola bar. Health-care practitioners need to start recommending bariatric surgery patients to consume simple whole foods and eat "real foods" instead of products with a nutrition label or ingredient statement.

Taparia and Koch describe the changes in food company formulations that are occurring as a result of consumer demand for removal of artificial colors and flavors, antibiotics in chicken, and emulsifiers like polyglycerol polyricinoleate in chocolate [22]. The food movement has been changing the food industry; soda sales have declined 25% since 1998 and orange juice sales have declined 45% since the juice became viewed as a source of free sugar stripped of natural fibers instead of as a healthy breakfast drink. The center aisles of the supermarket are still loaded with highly processed, high-sugar or high-fat food choices consumers need to reject.

Empowering individuals with the science of healing and well-being can do wonders pre- and postbariatric surgery. The alliance and collaboration among members of the health-care team is imperative to change food habits. Cheap food can be addictive and needs to become a controlled substance in the diet of bariatric surgery patients.

References

1. Nestle M. *Food Politics: How the Food Industry Influences Nutrition and Health.* Berkeley, CA: University of California Press. 2002.
2. Mercola J. How Junk Food Companies Have Hijacked Nutritional Science. Mercola.com, Nov 10, 2015.
3. Simon M. Nutrition: The scientists on the take from big food. Cornucopia Institute, Cornucopia, WI. Jul 1, 2015.
4. Poston WSC, Haddock CK, eds. *Food as a Drug.* New York, NY: The Haworth Press, 1999.
5. Schulte EA, Avena NM, Gearhardt AN. Which foods may be addictive? The role of processing, fat content, and glycemic load. *PLOS One* 2015 Feb 18;10(2):e0117959.
6. Mintz SW. *Sweetness and Power: The Place for Sugar in Modern History.* New York, NY: Penguin Books, 1985.
7. O'Connor A. Coca-Cola funds effort to alter obesity battle. *The New York Times,* Aug 10, 2015.
8. Pelchat ML, Johnson A, Chan R, et al. Images of desire: Food-craving activation during fMRI. *NeuroImage* 2004;23:1486–1493.
9. Roger PJ, Smit HJ. Food craving and food "addiction": A critical review of the evidence from a biopsychosocial perspective. *Pharm Biochem Behav* 2000;66:3–14.
10. Clemens R, Pressman P. Food craving: Signal of the heart, head or heritage? *Food Technol* 2005 Jul;59(7):21.
11. Bartelme MZ. No holds barred. *Food Technol* 2015 Feb;27–29.
12. Martindale D. Burgers on the brain: Can you really get addicted to fast food? *New Sci* 2003;177(2380):27–31.
13. McKenna P. Out of the trans-fat frying pan, into the fire. *New Sci* 2007;193(2585):13.
14. Watson A. Fast food sold at school lunch means more fat children. *San Jose Mercury News,* Mar 10, 2004.
15. Lipton KL, Edmondson W, Manchester A. *The Food and Fiber System: Contributing to the U.S. and World Economics.* Washington, DC: USDA Economic Research Service, 1998.
16. Gallo AE. *The Food Marketing System in 1996.* Washington, DC: USDA Economics Research Service 1998.
17. Kramer DE, Liston J, eds. *Seafood Quality Determination.* Amsterdam, the Netherlands: Elsevier Science Publishers, 1988.
18. Nettleton JA. *Seafood Nutrition: Facts, Issues and Marketing of Nutrition in Fish and Shellfish.* Huntington, NY: Osprey Books, 1983, p. 33.
19. Schneider A. Food Safety News, 2013. Available at: www .foodsafetynews.com.

20. Gardner R. Too Much Folic Acid in Vitamin Juices? Nutrition Outlook. Aug 29, 2014. Available at: http://www.nutritionaloutlook.com /vitamins-minerals/too-much-folic-acid-vitamin-juices.
21. Greenberg K. Coca-Cola Slammed for Deceptive Vitamin Water Marketing. Jan 16, 2009. Available at: Mediapost.com.
22. Taparia H, Koch P. Real food challenges the food industry. *The New York Times*, Nov 8, 2015.

2
PATHOPHYSIOLOGY OF OBESITY

Eat less and exercise more is the mantra for weight loss repeated by physicians, dietitians, and the food industry. It seems like such a simple equation: calories in – calories burned = weight management, but research does not support this outdated slogan.

Food choices have a greater influence on body metabolism than just calories. If you need 1,800 cal per day to maintain body weight and health and ate those 1,800 cal as French fries, your weight and health would not stay the same as eating 1,800 cal of lean meat and vegetables. Ingestion of high-fat, high-carbohydrate foods affect the central regulatory mechanisms for obesity management.

Sugar = Empty Calories

As Dr. John Yudkin, Professor of Nutrition and Dietetics at the University of London wrote in *Pure, White and Deadly* in 1986,

> More research has been done on the effects on health of the bread in our diet, or the eggs, or the breakfast cereals, or the meat, or the vegetables, than about the effects of sugar … what little research there had been already showed that sugar in the diet might be involved in the production of several conditions, including not only tooth decay and overweight but also diabetes and heart disease [1, pp. 1–2].

Dr. Yudkin points out, "There is no physiological requirement for sugar, all human nutritional needs can be met in full without having to take a single spoon of white or brown or raw sugar." He further comments in *Pure, White and Deadly*, "If only a small fraction of what is already known about the effects of sugar were to be revealed in relation to any other material used as a food additive, that material would promptly be banned" [1, p. 2].

Processed Foods = Obesity

By the twenty-first century, Holland and Petrovich were reporting on the addiction to a list of processed foods high in sugar, fat, and salt, which was a consequence of constant brain bombardment from all media that signaled leptin and insulin, and led to addictive behavior [2,3]. Those foods, associated with addictive behavior and activation of addictive responses in the brain, include chocolate, French fries, breakfast cereals, snack foods, sweet baked goods, dairy products, and pizza [4,5]. The evidence for addictive mechanisms related to highly processed foods crosses many types of research and needs further research so public health policy can begin to discuss the damage done by overeating.

Determining Body Fat Deposition

The body mass index (BMI) is still in use today as the means of assessing body adiposity despite the fact that it does not reflect the heterogeneity of fat deposition. Waist circumference (WC) is an important measure of adiposity since it relates better to an individual's health risk [6]. Some people store more of their excess fat viscerally, which increases WC. Research shows that fat distribution around the vital organs is a marker for insulin resistance and dyslipidemia. WC can complement the BMI in assessing morbidity. High risk is defined as a WC >40 in. (102 cm) for men and >35 in. (88 cm) for women [7].

Composition of Adipose Tissue

Normal body fat levels are considered to be a protective and insulating layer of fatty acids for body organs. Triglyceride storage in adipose tissue is the difference between energy consumed and energy needed for daily activities. The endocrine system controls the body fat storage signals through thyroid hormones, and the sympathetic and parasympathetic nervous systems [8]. Extra body fat in obese individuals causes the adipose tissue to create dysfunction in the immune system. Adipocytes can then produce lipid toxicity in other tissues [9, p. 21].

Lipids in cells serve two purposes—structure of cellular membrane and as fat storage depots. Fat depots are depleted during starvation to ensure membrane preservation. In the nonobese individual, body fat is approximately 15% body weight in males and 21% in females [9, p. 21]. Adipocytes are active in metabolism with both endocrine and paracrine functions [9, p. 22].

Those with higher BMIs are associated with greater percentages of body fat and increased leptin. A BMI >35 causes increased leptin, which should act as a negative regulator of body weight but instead has no effect in obesity [9, p. 23]. Elevated leptin levels in obese individuals are indicative of increased anorexigenic and decreased orexigenic peptide synthesis in the hypothalamus [10]. Leptin influences the hypothalamus through the signaling mechanism of neuropeptide Y and agouti-related protein, which stimulates eating similar to a cocaine–amphetamine transcription factor. Research into leptin functions in the body are ongoing, but it appears that leptin signals to the brain, the status of body fat stores, and failure of proper signaling are related to weight gain [11].

Another hormone, adiponectin, is derived from adipocytes and can lead to obesity-induced insulin resistance, cardiovascular events, and atherosclerosis [12]. Other secretory effects of adipokines include Interleukin 6 (IL-6), tumor necrosis factor (TNF), renin–angiotensin system, plasminogen activator inhibitor (PAI-1), adipsin (Complement D), and resistin [13].

Understanding Leptin

An overweight individual eating 2000 cal daily and not gaining weight decides to lose weight so that his knees and back do not hurt, or a physician has identified prediabetes and his patient is worried about having to take insulin. The individual initially loses a few pounds by reducing calorie intake, but as the leptin levels drop, the thyroid signals "starvation," which slows down the burning of fat and the weight loss stops [14].

The more frequently a person has repeated the lower calorie weight loss regime resulting in weight gain, the more leptin-resistance results. Once the person reaches a plateau and cannot lose any more weight, frustration leads to food-intake increase and leptin signals those calories to be stored as fat. Leptin is the survival hormone that enables humans to live for months with very little food.

As leptin causes the cell metabolism to slow down during any weight loss effort, it is also a factor that causes weight regain in bariatric surgery patients—particularly those candidates for adjustable gastric banding. Leptin problems are the cause of diet failures and the only solution for permanent weight loss is to learn how to master leptin levels [15].

- Allow 10–12 hours between the last meal of the day and breaking the fast (breakfast). Finish dinner/supper at least 3 hours before bed.
- Never go to bed on a full stomach.
- Eat at least three meals a day with 4–6 hours between meals. No snacking.
- Consume food slowly and in small amounts.
- Breakfast needs to contain a high-quality protein.
- Minimize carbohydrate foods.

Leptin levels follow a 24-hour natural cycle with peak levels in the evening and during the first hours of sleep. The lowest level of leptin is midday (noon to 1 PM) when it begins to gradually rise again. Obese individuals have lost their leptin rhythm [16, p. 120].

When leptin works properly, a high-leptin level controls the appetite and reduces the desire to eat [17]. People with leptin resistance have higher levels of leptin at night, but the brain does not receive the signal to control eating and individuals can raid the refrigerator or snack supply within hours after eating a large meal.

Bariatric surgery candidates with leptin resistance may also have insulin-resistance issues [16, p. 122]. Eating between meals leads to changes in hormonal signals that prevent the breakdown of fat. Insulin is released in response to an increase in blood glucose from the food consumed so that extra calories can be stored as fat. The first burst of insulin usually occurs within 10 minutes of eating with a peak around 30 minutes after a meal. The liver determines immediate energy needs and stores approximately 60% as glycogen for later use [18,19, pp. 8–9].

When muscles are not used enough to burn the glycogen, insulin facilitates storage of extra calories as fat. Insulin facilitates glucose entry into the fat cells where it is converted to glycerol to produce triglycerides [19, pp. 8–9]. Thus, high-insulin levels are a major reason calories are stored as fat and why fat cannot be broken down and used for energy.

Ghrelin

The gastrointestinal tract has a hormone called ghrelin that signals the hypothalamus in the brain to trigger hunger. The ghrelin hormone produced by the stomach rises when blood levels of leptin and glucose fall. High-fat diets also cause a rise in leptin and suppress ghrelin [20]. This hormone is essential for food emptying from the stomach into the small intestine.

In overweight individuals, ghrelin levels stay elevated after food is eaten, which causes excess consumption of food [21]. Ghrelin loses its normal rhythmic pattern for controlling eating behavior when leptin is too high. As leptin reduces, ghrelin levels can return to normal. Animal studies have shown that taking melatonin can decrease ghrelin levels [22].

Leptin and Thyroid

Leptin levels are a significant factor in metabolic rate because leptin controls thyroid function [23]. When leptin resistance occurs, the body thinks it is starving even with an overabundance of fat. The liver stops converting thyroid hormone (T4) into active thyroid hormone (T3) due to leptin resistance. Individuals with hypothyroid symptoms need to be assessed for leptin resistance.

Treatment Options

Treating obesity is similar to treating other chronic illnesses, according to Scott Kahan, MD, Director, National Center for Weight and Wellness, George Washington University, Washington, DC. He indicates that BMI, comorbidities, and patient preferences are important to the treatment plan.

Since obesity exists in world populations and all workplace environments, there are no quick fixes or universal options. Bariatric surgery is a tool to reduce food intake, but it needs to be part of a lifestyle change with cultural modifications in the work place and home.

Obesity defines a family and affects every member of the family while impacting the workplace and society. Excess body weight causes increased medical issues, depression, anxiety, decreased morale, and loss of productivity. Employers need to do more to reduce obesity by recognizing what employees eat and drink and encouraging a healthy lifestyle to offset the dangers of vending machines, microwave ovens, and food delivery options that contribute to obesity.

The increase in obesity is a difficult problem facing society today with little success from traditional methods of dieting and exercise. Bariatric surgery offers short-term success, but long-term benefits have yet to be tallied in personal health, medical costs, and quality of life. A meta-analysis of 11 studies reported that bariatric surgical patients lost more body weight and had higher remission rates for type 2 diabetes mellitus (T2DM) compared with nonsurgically managed patients [24].

Personalized treatment plans need to consider the following factors [25]:

Genetic factors like Prader–Willi syndrome, leptin pathway dysfunction, melanocortin 4 receptor gene

Epigenetics imprinting—DNA methylation and histone modifications, maternal obesity, excessive pregnancy weight gain

Environmental factors—high-calorie foods, sedentary behaviors, gut microbiota, stress, sleep patterns, medications

Hypothalmus regulation of energy—hunger, satiety, and energy compensation factors in metabolism

The World Health Organization (WHO) has recognized obesity as a disease and surgery as an option in weight management. Many patients are treated with lifestyle advice and appetite-suppressing drugs but the reality is that those with a BMI >40 are not likely to be successful without surgical treatment.

CASE STUDY 1

A case study of the traditional weight loss patient who cannot afford bariatric surgery but who wants to do something about his obesity follows.

LD is a 32-year-old Hispanic male, who has no insurance, who does not speak English, and who has two young children. He drives a delivery truck for a local bakery company.

Weight: 357 lb., BMI: 51.2, body fat: 45.8%.

LD denies eating anything all day until he gets home.

Cash price labs: complete blood count (CBC), comprehensive metabolic panel (CMP), thyroid panel completed.

Menu guide: Breakfast: low-sugar protein shake or egg sandwich; Lunch: Turkey Sandwich; Supper: chicken + small amount beans and rice, vegetable; Bedtime Snack: apple (NO sandwich as previously consumed).

One week later: Weight: 352 lb., BMI: 50.5. Lab review: Blood glucose (BG): 113, alanine aminotransferase (ALT): 47, thyroid-stimulating hormone (TSH): 1.46, free thyroxine (T4): 11.13, free triiodothyronine (T3): 3.6.

LD is unhappy he does not have a medical problem causing his weight gain. He proclaims he must have something wrong because he does not eat that much.

Cash pricing for carcinoembryonic antigen (CEA), cortisol, high-sensitivity C-reactive protein (hs-CRP). LD states he is hungry all night on diet.

Three weeks later, patient returns for lab review with entire family. Weight: 348 lb., BMI: 50, body fat: 45.7%. Labs: hs-CRP: 4.96, CEA: 1.0, cortisol: within normal limits.

LD is upset that he does not have cancer. He does not believe what he eats is the cause of his obesity. He is never seen again in the clinic.

References

1. Yudkin J. *Pure, White and Deadly*. London: Penguin Books. 1972, 1986.
2. Holland PC, Petrovich GD. A neural systems analysis of the potentiation of feeding by conditional stimuli. *Physiol Behav* 2005;86(5):747–761.

3. Corwin RL, Grigson PS. Food addiction: Fact or fiction symposium. *J Nutr* 2009; 139(3):617–619.
4. Harper TA, Mooney G. Prevention before profits: A levy on food and alcohol advertising. *Med J Austr* 2010;192(7):400–402.
5. Bagchi D, Preuss HG. *Obesity-Epidemiology, Pathophysiology, and Prevention*. Boca Raton, FL: CRC Press, 2013, pp. 59–60.
6. Tchernof A, Despres JP. Pathophysiology of human visceral obesity: An update. *Physiol Rev* 2013;93:359–404.
7. National Heart, Lung and Blood Institute, Obesity Education Initiative Expert Panel. Clinical guidelines on the identification, evaluation, and treatment of overweight and obesity in adults. The evidence report. *Obes Res* 1998;6 (Suppl 2):51S–209S.
8. Arone LJ, Mackintosh R, Rosenbaum M, et al. Autonomic nervous system activity in weight gain and weight loss. *Am J Physiol* 1995;269:R222.
9. Waine C, Bosanquet N. *Obesity and Weight Management in Primary Care*. Oxford, UK: Blackwell Science Ltd, 2002.
10. Reseland J, Anderssen SA, Solvoll K, et al. Effect of long-term changes in diet and exercise on plasma leptin concentrations. *Am J Clin Nutr* 2001;73(2):240–245.
11. Bluher M. Adipokines—Removing road blocks to obesity and diabetes therapy. *Mol Metab* 2014;3(3):230–240.
12. Flier JS, Spiegelman BM. Adipogenesis and obesity: Rounding out the big picture. *Cell* 1996;87:377–389.
13. McFarlane S, Banerji M, Sowers JR, et al. Insulin resistance and cardiovascular disease. *J Clin Endrocrinol Metab* 2001;86(2):713–718.
14. Ahima RS, Flier JS. Adipose tissue as an endocrine organ. *Trends Endocrinol Metab* 2000;11(8):327–332.
15. Trayhurn P, Hoggard N, Mercer JG, et al. Leptin: Fundamental aspects. *Int J Obesity* 1999;(23):22–28.
16. Richards BJ. *Mastering Leptin*. Minneapolis, MN: Wellness Resources Books, 2009.
17. Radic R, Nickolic V, Karner, I, et al. Circadian rhythm of blood leptin level in obese and non-obese people. *Coll Antropol* 2003 Dec;27(2):555–561.
18. Masuo K. Obesity-related hypertension: Role of the sympathic nervous system, insulin, and leptin. *Curr Hyperten Rep* 2002 Apr;4(2):112–118.
19. Powers MA. *Handbook of Diabetes Medical Nutritional Therapy*. Gaithersburg, MD: Aspen Publishers, 1996, pp. 8–9.
20. Caixas A, Bashore C, Nash W, et al. Insulin, unlike food intake, does not suppress ghrelin in human subjects. *J Clin Endocrinol Metab* 2002 Apr; 87(4):1902.
21. Bagnasco M, Kalra PS, Kalra SP, et al. Ghrelin and leptin pulse discharge in fed and fasted rats. *Endocrinology* 2002 Feb; 143(2):726–729.
22. Mustonen AM, Nieminen P, Hyvärinen H. Preliminary evidence of pharmacologic melatonin treatment decreases rat ghrelin levels. *Endocrine* 2001 Oct;16(1):43–46.

23. Guo F, Bakal K, Minokoshi Y, et al. Leptin signaling targets the thyrotropin-releasing hormone gene promoter in vivo. *Endocrinology* 2004 Feb 5;145(5):2221–2227.
24. Gloy VL, Briel M, Bhatt DL, et al. Bariatric surgery versus non-surgical treatment for obesity: A systematic review and meta-analysis of randomised controlled trials. *BMJ* 2013;347:f5934.
25. Bray G. *Handbook of Obesity. Classification and Evaluation of the Overweight Patient*. New York, NY: Marcel Dekker, Inc., 2004, pp. 1–32.

3

OVERVIEW OF BARIATRIC SURGERIES

Bariatric surgery is a medical procedure increasingly associated with long-term nutritional deficiencies that may have deleterious effects on each patient. The risks of malnutrition need to be evaluated in addition to comorbid disease concerns of coronary heart disease, diabetes mellitus, hypertension, hepatobiliary disease, endocrine abnormalities, malignancies, degenerative joint disease, cerebrovascular disease, respiratory abnormalities, and sudden death [1,2].

Psychosocial aspects of obesity can be a significant factor in selecting the surgical option for obesity management. Poor body image, low self-esteem, depression, and poor quality of life are frequently mentioned as the reasons for selecting bariatric surgery. Obesity is a chronic disease that according to the Centers for Disease Control and Prevention statistics, affects one-third of American adults (body mass index [BMI] >40) and another third are overweight (BMI >30) [3].

Reducing obesity through bariatric surgery can provide a sustainable weight-loss regime that numerous diets, meal substitutes, pills, exercise programs, behavior modification, hypnosis, and support groups have not been able to achieve with long-term success. Surgical therapy for weight loss has been controversial since its inception in the late 1950s, but recent refinements have decreased perioperative complications and reduced failure rates [4].

A January 2007 statistical review from the Agency for Healthcare Research and Quality reported that the total number of bariatric surgeries increased ninefold during 1998–2004—from 13,386 to 121,055 [5]. *Scientific American* reported that the average obese person costs society more than $7,000 per year in lost productivity and extra medical treatments, according to researchers at George Washington

University. Lifetime total medical costs for a person 70 lb. overweight were estimated at $30,000 [6]. Bariatric surgery remains the most effective way for lasting weight reduction and reducing medical costs.

Types of Bariatric Surgery

Early surgical procedures focused on limiting nutrient/calorie absorption. Kreman et al. produced weight loss through bypassing a significant portion of the intestines [7]. Other modifications eventually led to the Roux-en-Y gastroenterostomy with weight loss resulting from a small pouch partitioned from the stomach.

Roux-en-Y Gastric Bypass

Basic Description

- Restricts food volume and alters nutrient absorption
- Remission of type 2 diabetes mellitus (T2DM)
- Rapid improvement of blood glucose and blood pressure
- 50%–70% weight loss reported
- Dumping syndrome, vitamin and mineral deficiencies, constipation, vomiting
- Anemia, incisional hernia
- Intolerance to dairy

The Roux-en-Y gastric bypass (RYGB) surgery dramatically reduces the size of the stomach by producing a small pouch that receives food from the esophagus. The small intestine is cut at a point below the stomach and connected to the pouch creating a bypass for food around most of the stomach and part of the small intestine. The unused upper part of the small intestine that is connected to the bypassed stomach section is looped around and connected further down the small intestine creating a "Y" shape allowing gastric juices to drain.

Weight loss occurs from a combination of restriction on amount of food that can be eaten and changes in the neuronal and hormonal pathways. Most of the gastric bypass studies report weight loss in excess of the other procedures. Many individuals who lose weight rapidly from this procedure run the risk of gallstones and may need gallbladder removal during surgery to avoid complications.

Guidry et al. reported no significant difference in survival rates at 30 days and 1 year between patients with obesity undergoing gastric bypass surgery and those who did not chose the procedure [8].

The single anastomosis gastric bypass, also known as omega loop gastric bypass or mini-gastric bypass, has been increasing throughout Europe and Asia. Studies have labeled it a rapid, safe, and effective bariatric operation with expected weight loss compared with the RYGB. More information on the procedure can be found at the International Federation Surgery of Obesity website: ifso.com.

Vertical Sleeve Gastrectomy

Basic Description

- Restricts food volume and may decrease hormones that affect hunger
- Divides stomach vertically with 70%–85% of stomach permanently removed
- Cannot be converted to gastric bypass
- No intestinal rerouting
- 50%–60% weight loss reported
- Acid reflux
- Not reversible

Vertical sleeve gastrectomy (VSG) is becoming the surgery of choice for many surgeons and patients due to ease of surgery and elimination of bowel rearrangement with potential long-term complications. This procedure was first introduced in 1988 called a biliopancreatic diversion with duodenal switch (BPD-DS) [9]. Weight loss is achieved by limiting food portions and malabsorption mechanisms. The BPD is reported to exceed any other bariatric surgery for short- and long-term weight loss. Despite these good results, the numbers of BPD procedures have decreased, leaving the RYGB and VSG the most popular patient preference.

In the VSG procedure, 70%–85% of the stomach along the greater curvature is removed. The pylorus is retained and normal food grinding of the bolus enters the duodenal loop on its way to digestion and absorption. The sleeve resembles a long, thin banana whose size depends on the surgeon [10].

Increased problems with gastroesophageal reflux disease (GERD) have been associated with the sleeve, especially smaller sizes. A normal stomach can hold approximately 1,500 mL but the VSG reduces this volume to 90–220 mL.

The reduced stomach size causes early satiety and reduced oral intake, but increasing evidence suggests weight loss lifestyle modifications need to be made or else increased satiety from hormone changes can limit success. Studies have shown that when a sleeve is filled with saline the pressure inside rose to 43 mmHg compared with 34 mmHg when the stomach is intact. The surgery reduces the stomach's ability to distend causing fullness and reduced food intake.

Another aspect of appetite control in the VSG is the reduction of ghrelin-producing cells that are lost in the resecting and removal of most of the stomach [11]. Ghrelin is an endogenous hormone that stimulates the release of growth hormone and appetite. It plays a role in body weight regulation by initiating food intake. Ghrelin levels in VSG patients have been shown to remain low longer than 6 months postoperatively, which aids the weight loss process [12].

Laparoscopic sleeve gastrectomy is also gaining in popularity according to Young et al. because of lower morbidity with reduced blood loss, shorter operative time, and lower rate of deep wound infections [13].

The usual nutrient deficiencies of folate and vitamin D were identified by van Rutte et al. before and after sleeve gastrectomy [14], and Gehrer et al. reported fewer nutrient deficiencies from VSG than RYGB [15].

Stomach Intestinal Pylorus Sparing Surgery

Basic Description

- Slightly larger sleeve
- Attached to mid small intestine not distal ileum
- Preserves more bowel to prevent short bowel syndrome
- Ghrelin suppression
- Like VSG with intestinal shortening

Stomach intestinal pylorus sparing surgery (SIPS) is a modified duodenal switch surgery that reduces bowel issues like diarrhea while producing effective weight loss through reported management of ghrelin hormone reduction. It preserves the pyloric valve like the VSG and does not bypass as much of the intestine as the RYGB. Because it does not have a distal anastomosis and roux limb, it is believed to reduce long-term risk of intestinal obstruction and reduce gastrointestinal symptoms.

No increased risk of bile reflux gastritis is seen because the attachment is after the stomach valve. This procedure is considered as a solution for VSG patients who regain weight or have inadequate weight loss postoperatively.

Adjustable Gastric Banding

Basic Description

- Restricts food intake
- Adjustable band is reversible
- Less invasive procedure, faster recovery
- Modest weight loss 20%–25% initial weight (may be up to 40%)
- Foreign object in body (can be removed)
- Higher reoperation rate due to complications—band slippage or erosion

Adjustable gastric banding (AGB), also called LAP-BAND, is a fluid-filled belt wrapped around the stomach to create an upper pouch that receives food from the esophagus while the lower pouch drains into the small intestine. A tube leads from the belt to a port just under the surface of the abdomen. Through the port, the physician can either add or remove fluid from the belt to adjust its tightness. The tightness of the belt regulates how easily food moves between the stomach's upper and lower pouches.

In 2011, a Food and Drug Administration advisory panel voted to allow those with BMIs >30 or more, rather than the minimum BMI >35 to apply for gastric banding weight loss surgery. They must have tried and failed more traditional weight loss therapies—diet, exercise, and appetite suppression medications. The study was initiated and supported by Allergan, a maker of the laparoscopic adjustable gastric band (LAP-BAND) system procedure [16].

LAP-BAND is a purely restrictive procedure to control food intake. It has a low mortality rate and allows gradual weight loss. The AGB procedure is a good choice for those with regular exercise programs and disciplined food choices. Adjustments can be done every 4–8 weeks in the physician's office, which is important in case of pregnancy.

Although patients lose weight, many regain some or all of the lost weight by overeating soft foods (i.e., ice cream) or smoothies made from high-carbohydrate and fatty foods. Since there is no modification in absorption, food discipline is critical for success. Lifelong vitamin and nutritional supplementation is still recommended to insure adequate intake of proteins, B vitamins, calcium, and trace minerals.

Gastric band slippage is a challenge that can affect weight loss and cause dysphagia and pain [17]. Slippage frequently requires revision surgery. Poor postoperative compliance with diet restrictions have been linked to band slippage [18] and disparity in dietary instructions [19] can result in deleterious results.

Benefits of Bariatric Surgery

Research has shown that mitochondrial disorders from adipose tissue leading to T2DM have been improved with RYGB but those choosing a less aggressive weight loss surgery will not get the same benefit. Jahansouz et al. reported lack of improvement in glycemic control and mitochondrial function following AGB [20].

But bariatric surgery remains more effective for lasting weight loss than dieting and exercise. The first year after surgery can be a "honeymoon" with new food choices, new habits, and improved self-esteem but many patients soon start regaining weight. Dr. John Morton, past president of the American Society for Metabolic and Bariatric Surgery (ASMBS) and head of bariatric surgery at Stanford University School of Medicine, California, indicates that obese patients who regain some weight can still see health benefits from the surgery [21].

Peter T. Hallowell, MD, of the University of Virginia, Department of Surgery, Charlottesville, Virginia, and colleagues studied bariatric surgery in 401 patients and reported a clear survival advantage in morbidly obese patients who pursued gastric bypass surgery over those not undergoing the procedure [22].

Benefits of bariatric surgery can also be considered for adolescents who do not lose weight despite increased physical activity and better food choices. Individuals at least 16 years old and those with a BMI >40 may be considered for surgical intervention to offset further obesity challenges. Since weight loss surgery curbs the sweet tooth by acting on the brain's reward system, younger obese patients may find the surgery more effective than traditional programs [23].

Other Bariatric Surgery Considerations

According to Dr. Andrei Keidar and colleagues at Tel Aviv University, much needs to be learned about patient selection for surgery to enhance long-term success. They followed 443 obese patients who had VSG to see how much weight they lost and what improvements in health they experienced. After 1 year, participants had averaged a loss of 77% of their original weight. But in 5 years, many participants had only retained a weight loss of 56% of their original weight. Participants in the study had significantly reduced low-density lipoprotein (LDL) cholesterol levels in 1 year and 3 years, but little change by the fifth year [24].

Shikora et al. reported that many investigators attribute failures in bariatric surgery to patient noncompliance. After surgery, patients are advised to adhere to strict dietary guidelines but some patients ignore the restrictions, which leads to pouch dilatation, stomal enlargement, and staple disruption. A few patients have been reported to consume high-calorie drinks that cause inadequate weight loss [4].

Ethnicity may affect the success of bariatric surgery since some studies have reported better weight loss among non-Hispanic whites versus non-Hispanic blacks and Hispanics [25]. Weight loss and BMI reduction was similar among non-Hispanic whites and Hispanics compared with non-Hispanic blacks who had gastric bypass surgery. No significant ethnic difference was noted for AGB patients.

Gender is another potential factor that can influence weight loss after surgery. Bekheit et al. reported gastric banding to be less effective in males [26] but Perrone et al. concluded males had greater BMI loss than females post-VSG and RYGB surgeries [27].

Age appears to be less of a factor in patient selection for bariatric surgery although Abbas et al. indicated long-term effects need further studies. Their study indicated patients older than 60 were safe and effective candidates with low morbidity and mortality [28].

A good surgical result does not ensure a successful weight loss. Surgery is only one aspect in the management of obesity. Nutrition management pre- and postsurgery is needed to maximize weight loss, food avoidance, behavior change, improved physical activity, and compliance in nutrient supplementation.

CASE STUDY 1

RS, a 69-year-old male, had RYGB followed 3 days later with kinked bowel surgery and subsequent surgeries for hiatal hernia and small bowel blockage requiring mesh screen within 3 months post-RYGB. Presurgery weight: 294 lb. His cardiologist recommended surgery to be able to see his grandchildren grow up.

Weight on first nutrition consult 2 years post-RYGB: 112.4 lb., body mass index (BMI): 16.6, body fat: 8.6%.

RX: Pepcid, primidone, warfarin, amiodipine, sertraline.

Labs: Methylenetetrahydrofolate reductase (*MTHFR*): AC heterozygous, high-sensitivity C-reactive protein (hs-CRP): 3.8, homocysteine: 12, hemoglobin (Hgb): 12.4, albumin (Alb): 3.5, thyroid-stimulating hormone (TSH): 1.4, thyroxine (T4): 6.9, triiodothyronine (T3): 146, vitamin D: 15, amylase and lipase: within normal limits (WNL).

SX: Failure to thrive.

Plan of Care: Oral nutrient supplementation: amino acids, basic multiple vitamin and mineral, probiotics, folate, medium-chain triglycerides (MCT) oil. Intramuscular (IM) injection of 50,000 IU 25-hydroxy vitamin D_3 (25-OH Vit D3). Bariatric postsurgery ketogenic diet. Intravenous (IV) nutrition repletion 2 weeks × 4 weeks (ascorbic acid, B vitamins, magnesium, zinc).

One month later: Weight: 116, BMI: 17.1, body fat: 8.4% (Monolaurin [lauric acid] supplement for travel). Labs: Cholesterol: 175, triglycerides: 54, hs-CRP: 4.5, vitamin D: 39, hemoglobin/hematocrit (H/H): 11/34. IV nutrition continued weekly.

Two months later: Weight: 116.6, BMI: 17.2, body fat: 8.4%. Add ribose for energy + extra fat in food choices and preparation. IM 50,000, IU 25-OH Vit D3. Begin IM daily B complex + B_{12} shots. Recommend testosterone for libido and stamina.

Three months later: Weight: 118, BMI: 17.4, body fat: 9.1%. Increase probiotics for bowel improvement. Diet review—add variety in food choices. Labs: H/H: 13.4/40.5, blood glucose (BG): 122 (nF), hs-CRP: 0.5, vitamin D: 57.

Four months later: Weight: 123.8, BMI: 18.3, body fat: 9.4%. Testosterone patches started. Diet includes bowl of ice cream HS to take nutrition supplements. Spectra Cell Laboratory Nutrition Testing: deficient in oleic acid and vitamin A.

Five months later: Weight: 127, BMI: 18.8, body fat: 9.6%. IV nutrition for viral management per lab testing. Added nutrition supplements lipoic acid and lysine. Testosterone IM monthly × 3 to replace patches. Set weight gain goals + reviewed dietary food choices to continue healthy weight management. Each nutrition counseling session focuses on his excellent compliance to nutrition supplementation and his ongoing need.

CASE STUDY 2

WMC, a 46-year-old female 7 years post-AGB who previously worked night shift but is now disabled with hypertension and constant pain. She is scheduled for RYGB. First pregnancy weight: 180 lb., second pregnancy weight: 205 lb., third pregnancy weight: 250 lb., and "hungry all 9 months." Current weight: 489 lb., BMI: >61.

24-Hour food intake: Breakfast: milk shake; Lunch: bologna and cheese sandwich, peach, or apple; Dinner: pizza and fried chicken + soda.

Nutrition consultation—helped patient modify food intake but she continued to describe poor sleep pattern and severe pain in knees. After much focus on food choices as it is important in RYGB surgery, patient was still only interested in how much weight she needed to lose so she could have knee surgery.

References

1. Bray GA. Complications of obesity. *Ann Inter Med* 1985; 103:1052–1062.
2. Van Itallie TB. Obesity: Adverse effects on health and longevity. *Am J Clin Nutr* 1979; 32:2723.
3. Center for Disease Control and Prevention. *Overweight and Obesity: Obesity Trends: U.S. Obesity Trends.* Washington, DC: Center for Disease Control and Prevention 2005, pp. 1985–2004.
4. Shikora SA, Benotti PN, Forse RA. Surgical treatment of obesity. In: Blackburn GL, Kanders BS, eds. *Obesity Pathophysiology Psychology and Treatment.* New York, NY: Chapman & Hall, 1994, pp. 264–272.
5. Zhao Y, Encinosa W. Bariatric Surgery Utilization and Outcome in 1998 and 2004. Available at: www.hcup-us.ahrq.gov.reports/statbriefs.
6. Freedman DH. A plan to fix the obesity crisis. *Scientific Amer special ed* 2015;24:2.
7. Kreman AJ, Linner JH, Nelson CH. An experimental evaluation of the nutritional importance of proximal and distal small intestine. *Ann Surg* 1954;140:439–448.
8. Guidry CA, Davies SW, Sawyer RG, et al. Gastric bypass improves survival compared with propensity-matched controls: A cohort study with over 10-year follow-up. *Am J Surg* 2015;209:463–467. doi 10.1016/j.amjsurg.2014 10.009.
9. Brethauer SA, Hammel JP, Schauer PR. Systemic review of sleeve gastrectomy staging and primary bariatric procedure. *Surg Obes Relat Dis* 2009;5:469–75.
10. Shi X, Karmali S, Sharma AM, et al. A review of laparoscopic sleeve gastrectomy for morbid obesity. *Obes Surg* 2010;20:1171–1177.
11. Bueter M, le Roux CW. Gastrointestinal hormones, energy balance and bariatric surgery. *Int J Obes* (Lond) 2011;35:S35–39.
12. Peterli R, Steinert R, Woelnerhanssen B, et al. Metabolic and hormonal changes after laparoscopic Roux-en-Y gastric bypass and sleeve gastrectomy: A randomized prospective trial. *Obes Surg* 2012;22:740–748.
13. Young MT, Gebhart A, Phelan MJ, et al. Use and outcomes of laparoscopic sleeve gastrectomy vs laparoscopic gastric bypass: Analysis of the American College of Surgeons NSQIP. *J Amer Coll Surg* 2015; 220:880–885.
14. van Rutte PWJ, Aarts EO, Smulders JF, et al. Nutrient deficiencies before and after sleeve gastrectomy. *Obes Surg* 2014; 24:1639–1646.
15. Gehrer S, Kern B, Peters T, et al. Fewer nutrient deficiencies after laparoscopic sleeve gastrectomy (LSG) than after laparoscopic Roux Y gastric bypass (LRYGB)—A prospective study. *Obes Surg* 2010;20:447–453.
16. Peck P, Ex Ed. FDA Expands Gastric Band Indication. *Med Page Today.* Feb 16, 2011.
17. Findlay L, Ball W, Ramus J. Gastric band slippage: The impact of a change in education and band filling. *Obes Surg* 2015;25:1302–1306.

18. Suter M. Laparoscopic band repositioning for pouch dilatation/slippage after gastric banding patients eating 1 year post surgery? *Obes Surg* 2012;22(12):507–512.

19. Mc Grice MA, Porter JA. What are gastric banding patients eating 1 year post surgery? *Obes Surg* 2012;22 (12):1855–1858.

20. Jahansouz C, Serrot FJ, Frohnert BI, et al. Roux-en-Y gastric bypass acutely decreases protein carbonylation and increases expression of mitochondrial biogenesis genes in subcutaneous adipose tissue. *Obes Surg* 2015;25:2376–2385.

21. Wolfe BM, Morton J. Weighing in on bariatric surgery: Procedure use, readmission rates, and mortality. *JAMA.* 2015; 204(15): 1960-1963.

22. Hallowell PT. Endocrine Today, March 2015.

23. Han W, Tellez LA, Niu J, et al. Striatald dopamine links gastrointestinal rerouting to altered sweet appetite. *Cell Metab* 2016;23(1):103–112.

24. Rapaport L. Benefits of weight loss surgery diminish after 5 years. *Scientific Amer* 2015 Aug 5. Available at: http://www.scientificamerican .com/article/benefits-of-weight-loss-surgery-diminish-after-5-years/.

25. Khorgami Z, Arheart KL, Zhang C, et al. Effect of ethnicity on weight loss after bariatric surgery. *Obes Surg* 2015;25:769–776.

26. Bekheit M, Katri K, Ashour MH, et al. Gender influences on long-term weight loss after three bariatric procedures: Gastric banding is less effective in males in a retrospective analysis. *Surg Endosc* 2014;28(8):2406–2411.

27. Perrone F, Bianciardi E, Benavoli D, et al. Gender influence on long-term weight loss and comorbidities after laparoscopic sleeve gastrectomy and Roux-en-Y gastric bypass: A prospective study with a 5-year follow-up. *Obes Surg* 2016; 26(2): 276–281.

28. Abbas M, Cumella L, Zhang Y, et al. Outcomes of laparoscopic sleeve gastrectomy and roux-en-y gastric bypass in patients older than 60. *Obes Surg* 2015;25:2251–2256.

4

NUTRITION ASSESSMENT

Long-term success of bariatric surgery begins with a comprehensive nutrition assessment designed to evaluate signs and symptoms related to the obesity problem unique to the individual. A food and nutrition history of eating habits, weight history, and family-related medical issues helps identify counseling needs for eating behavior changes and attitude about dietary supplement use.

Anthropometric measurements are needed to assess the diagnosis and treatment options. A presurgery diet for modifying portions and food choices—ketogenic low-carbohydrate diet, Mediterranean or dietary approaches to stop hypertension (DASH) diet, or low-glycemic diet—assists the candidate in preparing for surgery. A dietary supplementation regime helps bariatric surgery patients replete themselves with nutrients prior to surgery and develops a regular habit of supplementation intake postsurgery.

Assessment

Objective measures of nutrition health are critical to determine a candidate's understanding of nutrition requirements pre- and postsurgery. These include the following:

- Anthropometric measurements
- Daily food habits or diet history
- Medication and dietary supplement intake
- Medical history
- Weight history
- Clinical nutrition examination
- Psychological support
- Physical activity

Since biochemical assessments are usually not available, past medical history information regarding anemia, dyslipidemia, and blood glucose management needs to be obtained during the assessment.

Anthropometric Measurements

Anthropometric measurements include body weight, height, percentage of body fat, and body mass index (BMI), which is the weight in kilograms divided by height in meters squared (BMI= kg/m^2) [1]. Excess body fat contributes to increased morbidity and mortality and BMI values can help motivate the candidate to change diet and lifestyle habits. Waist circumference can be useful in evaluating the success of weight loss treatments and is a better predictor of disease risk than BMI for persons of Asian descent and in the elderly for estimating obesity-related disease risk [1, p. 189].

Interest in body composition data has increased in the past decade due to the rising level of obesity. Estimating fat and protein reserves is an important aspect of the nutrition assessment. Various methods are available for estimating body fat and muscle mass—skin fold measurements, underwater weighing, air displacement plethysmography, and electrical impedance [1, pp. 204–210]. A general guide to BMI levels is as follows:

<20—potential for nutritional deficiencies
20–26—desirable
27–29—moderately overweight
>30—obese

Diet History

Nutrition evaluation through the review of a 24-hour food recall or diet history provides an overview of what and how much food and nutrition education needs to be included. A three-step approach can be used in obtaining a diet history. Step one is to collect general information about food habits that have contributed to weight gain. Step two is questioning the individual about their usual eating pattern, and step three is to cross check the accuracy of information in step two by repeating the questions about the previous day's meals.

During the assessment, the nutritionist questions the number of meals eaten per day, food likes and dislikes, and any food allergies or sensitivities in an effort to become familiar with the candidate. Estimates of protein intake can be made in an effort to customize the assessment to the required protein and nutrient needs postsurgery. Individuals with recall problems need a spouse or caregiver to be present and/or available to provide appropriate data. Those with impaired vision or hearing may need an interpreter, and those who are reading impaired or have language difficulties need additional technology devices for learning. Food models can be useful in helping estimate portions.

Use of vitamin and mineral supplements and other over-the-counter products can provide an insight into the discussion on nutrition supplementation, which will be needed postsurgery.

An individual's ability to chew and swallow needs to be assessed in the interview. Natural teeth or dentures that fit well will be needed to provide good mastication postsurgery. Poor-fitting dentures and missing teeth may be critical to their nutrition adequacy postsurgery.

Alcohol use and medications need to be reviewed during the assessment drug–nutrient interactions can have adverse effects on the candidate's status pre- and postsurgery such as the following:

- High alcohol intake = loss of protein + thiamine, niacin, and folate deficiency
- Statin drugs = Coenzyme Q_{10} needs
- Antacids = Vitamin B_{12} loss
- Cigarette smoking = Vitamin C and folate insufficency

Medical History

Essential components of a candidate's medical history are gathered during the nutrition assessment because they may impact current and postsurgery health [2].

Cardiovascular risk factors like dyslipidemia, hypertension, and diabetes mellitus are associated with dietary factors.

Congestive heart failure—thiamine deficiency
Cardiomyopathy—selenium deficiency
Rapid heart rate—thiamine deficiency
Hyperhomocysteinemia—folate, vitamin B_{12}, vitamin B_6 deficiency

Pulmonary strength can be diminished by protein calorie malnutrition and this leads to chronic disorders like chronic obstructive pulmonary disease (COPD).

Gastrointestinal disorders may result from food sensitivities, medications, or gluten sensitivity.

Inflammatory bowel disease—protein calorie malnutrition
Liver disease—protein calorie malnutrition
Pancreatic insufficiency—vitamins D, A, E, A deficiency
Atrophic gastritis—vitamin B_{12} deficiency

Musculoskeletal issues can influence weight loss potential and quality of life postsurgery.

Generalized muscle weakness/endurance—dehydration, iron deficiency, nutrient deficiencies
Muscle wasting—vitamin D, protein calorie deficiency
Osteoporosis—Calcium, magnesium, vitamin D

Thyroid disorders can be assessed by physical examination of reflex time, basal body temperatures and laboratory testing of thyroid stimulating hormone (TSH), free triiodothyronine (T3), free thyroxine (T4), reverse T3, and thyroid peroxidase (TPO) antibodies.

Clinical Nutrition Examination

Common nutritional disorders can be assessed by close examination of skin, nails, mouth, and eyes [3].

Skin
Dermatitis—vitamin B_6, zinc
Impaired wound healing—vitamin C, zinc, protein
Rash (arms, legs)—niacin
Bruising—vitamin K_1
Dry flaky skin—essential fatty acids, vitamin A
Depigmentation—protein calorie malnutrition
Pallor—iron, vitamin B_{12}, folate
Nails
Spoon-shaped—iron deficiency
Discolored—selenium toxicity
Ridged—protein calorie malnutrition

Hair

Discoloration, dullness, loss—protein calorie malnutrition

Alopecia—biotin deficiency

Eyes

Poor night vision—vitamin A

Oral

Swollen, bleeding gums—vitamin C

Bones and Joints

Beading ribs, bowlegs—vitamin D

Neurological

Disorientation—thiamine

Peripheral neuropathy—thiamine, vitamin B_6, vitamin B_{12}

Psychosocial Support

Reviewing the bariatric surgery candidate's age, occupation, educational level, marital status, income, living arrangements, and dependents provides a more complete snapshot of how to proceed with the nutrition education needed for success postsurgery.

Physical Activity

Epidemiological studies suggest that physical inactivity is a major cause of obesity. There is little agreement that a sedentary lifestyle is the cause of obesity or that physical activity prevents weight gain through improved metabolic management. The evidence to support a more active lifestyle as the key to weight loss and improved health is weak [4] so a modest approach to increased walking, biking, or swimming could help improve weight loss potential with a 30-minute per day recommendation. A combination of surgery-induced diet restrictions and modest daily exercise may be the key to future success but more research is needed on this.

Drug–Nutrient Interactions

Clinicians can fail to recognize the importance of drug–nutrient interactions when assessing the nutrition status of bariatric surgery patients but health-care professionals need to be aware of the malnutrition factors that drugs may cause. Medications may modify nutrient absorption, metabolism, and excretion of nutrients in the following ways:

- Alter nutrient absorption by changing the acidity of the digestive tract (e.g., antacids interfere with iron and folate absorption)
- Damage the small intestine mucosal cells
- Bind nutrients (e.g., bile acid binders bind to fat-soluble vitamins)
- Stimulate gastric acid secretion (e.g., antifungal ketoconazole is absorbed better with meals due to acid secretion)
- Alter gastric emptying (e.g., when drugs are taken with food)
- Compete with food for absorption in the intestines, especially amino acids
- Use similar enzyme systems for metabolism (e.g., liver enzymes increase metabolism of folate, vitamin D, vitamin K)
- Alter reabsorption in kidneys (e.g., diuretics increase excretion of sodium and potassium) [5]

Drugs and nutrients interact metabolically because they use the same enzyme systems in the small intestines and liver. Drugs may enhance or inhibit the activity of enzymes needed for normal nutrient metabolism or dietary components may enhance or inhibit enzymes that break down drugs. Select examples include [5] the following:

- Methotrexate—used for inflammation, resembles folate, and competes with the enzyme that converts folate into its active form
- Corticosteroids—used for inflammation and immunosuppression can cause weight gain, muscle wasting, bone loss, hyperglycemia
- Phenobarbital and phenytoin—used as anticonvulsant interferes with the metabolism of vitamins D and K
- Warfarin—used as anticoagulant interacts with vitamin K to prevent blood-clotting factors

- Monoamine oxidase (MAO) inhibitors—medications used to treat depression block an enzyme that inactivates tyramine, epinephrine, and norepinephine

The enzyme system responsible for the metabolism of most nutrients and drugs is the cytochrome P450 (CYP) enzyme family located in the endoplasmic reticulum of the hepatocytes and enterocytes [6]. Vitamins and dietary factors are known to modify CYP activity. Dietary factors that increase CYP activity are

- Calorie restriction
- Charcoal cooked foods
- Garlic oil, fish oil
- Protein supplementation
- Thiamine deficiency
- Vitamin E supplementation

Dietary factors that reduce CYP activity are

- Iron deficiency
- Protein deficiency
- Starvation
- Vitamin A deficiency
- Vitamin C deficiency

Failure to identify and manage drug–nutrient interactions can cause serious consequences like compromised immune function, treatment failure, or morbidity [6].

Drugs that are recommended to be taken with food to maximize absorption are [7,8]

Albendazole	Ketoconazole
Amiodarone	Lithium
Atazanavir	Lopinavir
Atovaquone	Lovastatin
Cefuroxime	Mefloquine
Erythromycin	Nelfinavir
Ganciclovir	Rifapentine
Griseofulvin	Ritonavir
Hydralazine	Saquinavir

Drugs that should not be taken with food to allow optimal absorption are [7,9,10]

Ampicillin	Isoniazid
Captopril	Norfloxacin
Ciprofloxacin	Oflaxacin
Didanosine	Rifampin
Dicloxacillin	Voriconazole
Doxycycline	Zafirlukast
Indinavir	

The reason for not consuming drugs with food include: acid liability, chelation, or binding with food content.

Drug–Nutrient Issues Frequently Seen in Bariatric Surgery Patients

- Acid-suppression therapy: histamine blockers and proton pump inhibitors (PPI) inhibit absorption of vitamin B_{12} from food and decrease iron and beta-carotene absorption [11].
- Amitriptyline for depression depletes vitamin B_6 [11].
- Angiotensin-converting enzyme (ACE) inhibitors for hypertension deplete zinc [11].
- Antibiotics reduce microbiota so probiotics are needed during therapy and 1–2 weeks after treatment is completed [11].
- Aspirin increases urinary excretion of vitamin C [11].
- Beta-blockers inhibit coenzyme Q_{10} [11].
- Calcium-channel blockers for hypertension have greater bioavailability when taken with grapefruit juice [11].
- Colchicine decreases vitamin B_{12} absorption [11].
- Contraceptives (oral) cause vitamin B_6 deficiency, folate deficiency, vitamin B_{12}, thiamine, and riboflavin insufficiency [11].
- Cyclosporine causes hypomagnesemia. Ingestion of red wine reduces bioavailability of cyclosporine [11].
- Diuretics increase urinary excretion of potassium, magnesium, chloride, zinc [11].
- Fluoroquinolones bind magnesium, calcium, iron, zinc, manganese. Do not take mineral containing supplements within 1–2 hours before or 2–6 hours after the drug dose [11].

- Levothyroxine is inhibited by calcium carbonate, iron, magnesium oxide, and soy protein [11].
- Metformin inhibits vitamin B_{12} absorption [11].
- Statin absorption is increased when consumed with grapefruit juice so consumption of grapefruit juice is not recommended and pomegranate juice needs to be avoided because it inhibits P_{450} enzyme. Statins decrease coenzyme Q_{10} levels in plasma and muscle [11].

Nutrition Education

The effectiveness of the nutrition assessment and counseling session is based on the adequacy of the interview process and communication skills of the educator. The dietary counseling process will be most effective when the nutritionist does not evaluate diet habits but provides **new** guidelines in an effort to minimize defensiveness about habits that contributed to weight gain. Each person knows they need to change lifestyle habits but encouragement and support for the change will be more effective than judging previous mistakes [12].

Instead of judging poorly controlled diabetes, a better approach is to discuss which foods in the diet need to be changed or reduced. An example from the author's experience over 20 years ago is telling an obese patient that "they were being irresponsible" because they ate a whole box of chocolates instead of one or two pieces. The patient went back to the physician complaining about, "how judgmental I was and never wanted to see me again."

A person-centered approach to nutrition counseling advocated by Carl Rogers, PhD [13,14] needs to be the norm for helping obese individuals adjust to new guidelines for a healthier life. Behavior modification with self-monitoring and record keeping of a diet and weight journal can increase counselor–patient interaction, which allows a better self-monitored behavior for long-term success [15]. Unfortunately, insurance companies require only one nutrition counseling session for the patient prior to surgery and nothing postsurgery when behavior changes are most critical.

Presurgery Eating Goals

Presurgery eating habits need to focus on increasing intake of nutrient-dense foods that provide essential nutrients but are relatively low in calories. Nutrient-dense foods include: broccoli, spinach, carrots, baked potato, turkey, chicken, fish, plain yogurt, and fresh fruit. Low-nutrient foods include: French fries, fast-food burgers, hot dogs, fruit-flavored yogurt, sweetened sodas, and juices.

Dietary consumption goals need to focus on decreasing simple carbohydrates, limiting high-sodium foods and reducing portion sizes. A sample menu guide should be provided for presurgery and postsurgery during the nutrition assessment so the individual recognizes the total dietary modifications needed for successful weight loss. An example of a presurgery bariatric menu is as follows:

Presurgery Bariatric Menu—Learning Portion Control

Breakfast Menu Ideas

2 oz. protein or 2 scoops whey protein powder (14–15 g protein)

2 scrambled eggs + 6 fresh large strawberries

or

2 oz. lean turkey sausage + 1/2 cup frozen mango cubes

or

Banana smoothie: 1/4 cup plain full fat yogurt, 2 scoops protein powder, 1/2 banana, 3 ice cubes. Blend until smooth

Lunch Menu Ideas

2–3 oz. protein, 1 or more vegetables, 1 starch, 1 fat

3 oz. chopped chicken (leftover from dinner) + 2 cups mixed salad greens + 2 tablespoons Ranch or Italian dressing and 1/2 cup potato salad

or

3 oz. flaked tuna + 1 tablespoon mayo on 1 slice bread covered with 1 oz. mozzarella cheese. Broil and cut into 4 pieces. Eat with carrot, celery, cherry tomatoes

or

6 large or 12 medium cooked shrimp, cocktail sauce + 6 oz. low-sodium V8 juice and 4 rice crackers with 1 oz. goat cheese

Dinner Menu Ideas

2–3 oz. protein, 1 or more vegetables, 1 starch or fruit, 1 fat

3 large sea scallops sauteed in 1 tablespoon butter + 1/2 cup steamed spinach and 2 small red potatoes

or

3 oz. turkey sausage in 1/4 cup marinara sauce + 1/2 cup basmati rice and 1/2 cup peas and carrots with 1 teaspoon butter

or

3 oz. baked salmon with 1 cup mixed greens with 1 tablespoon dressing + 1/2 cup steamed green beans and 1/2 cup fresh fruit and 2 tablespoons plain yogurt

Snacks

1 oz. protein + 1 starch or fat or fruit

1/4 cup guacamole + 1 scoop protein powder + raw vegetables (carrots, celery, cucumber slices)

or

1/4 cup cottage cheese + 1/2 cup frozen berries

References

1. Lee RD, Nieman DC. *Nutrition Assessment*. New York, NY: McGraw-Hill, 2012, pp. 170–210.
2. Hensrud DD. Nutrition screening and assessment. *Med Clin N Amer* 1999;83:1525–1546.
3. Coulson AM, Rock CL, Monsen ER, eds. *Nutrition in the Prevention and Treatment of Disease*. New York, NY: Academic Press, 2001, p. 49.
4. Rissanen A, Fogelholm M. Physical activity in the prevention and treatment of other morbid conditions and impairments associated with obesity: Current evidence and research issues. *Med Sci Sports Exerc* 1999;31:S635–S645.
5. Rolfes SR, Pinna K, Whitney E, eds. *Understanding Normal and Clinical Nutrition*. Belmont, CA: Thomson-Wadsworth, 2006, p. 635.
6. Shils ME, Shike M, Ross AC, et al. *Modern Nutrition in Health and Disease*. Baltimore, MD: Lippincott Williams & Wilkins, 2006, p. 1547.
7. Schmidt LE, Dalhoff K. Food-drug interactions. *Drugs* 2002;62:1481–502.
8. Orrick JJ, Steinhart CR. Atazanavir. *Ann Pharmacother* 2004;38:1664–74.

9. Burman WJ, Gallicano K et al. *Clin Pharmacol* 2003;56[Suppl 1]:17–23.

10. Purkins L, Wood N, Kleinermans D, et al. Effect of food on the pharmacokinetics of multiple-dose oral voriconazole. *Br J Clin Pharmacol* 2003;56[Suppl 1]:17–23.

11. Gaby AR. *Nutritional Medicine.* Concord, NH: Fritz Perlberg Publishing, 2011, pp. 1305–1317.

12. Bauer KD, Sokolik CA. *Basic Nutrition Counseling Skill Development.* Belmont, CA: Wadsworth/Thomson Learning, 2002.

13. Rogers C. *On Becoming a Person: A Therapist's View of Psychotherapy.* Boston, MA: Houghton Mifflin, 1961.

14. Rogers C. *Carl Rogers on Personal Power: Inner Strength and Its Revolutionary Impact.* New York. NY: Delacorte, 1977.

15. Stunkard AJ, Berthold HC. What is behavioral therapy? A very short description of behavioral weight control. *Am J Clin Nutr* 1985;41:821–823.

5

SETTING NUTRITION GOALS FOR BARIATRIC PATIENTS

Bariatric surgery is an effective weight loss option for obese individuals [1] and health-care professionals are critical in helping them set nutritional goals for successful weight loss and healthy lifestyle habits. The individual cost of being obese is $4,879 and $2,646 for women and men, respectively, according to the George Washington University School of Public Health Services Department of Health Policy [2]. The analysis demonstrates that costs are nine times higher for women and six times higher for men in work-related costs like lost wages, absenteeism, and disability. No research has offered insight into consumer costs such as clothing, air travel, automobile size, and furniture expenditures.

Lifestyle modifications are needed by every obese patient with nutrition as a cornerstone for management. No single diet has proven to be superior in terms of weight loss, and bariatric surgery modifications need to be personalized to the individual for efficacy in weight reduction [3]. As Parker et al. state, individuals with presurgery eating pathology are more likely to retain disordered eating behaviors after surgery and experience poorer weight loss and more physical health complications [4].

The challenge is to diagnose and change eating habits prior to surgery. Candidates for bariatric surgery need to understand that weight reduction in the United States is a $30 billion business consisting of dietary supplements, diet foods, new exercise regimens, and cleanses. Since these are not individualized the solutions may produce some weight loss but it is quickly regained because attitudes and choices are not changed [5].

Candidates need to prepare for surgery as if their life depends on it. That includes retraining the brain and understanding that exercise does not come in a pill. As Americans watch more food shows on television, and eat more processed foods at restaurants or at home, so has their waistline increased. Devouring a 1,000 cal fast food meal in

10 minutes does not allow enough time for stomach signals from the first bite to turn off a hunger hormone in the brain.

Obesity is directly related to our present day modern diet. Grain cultivation marked the time when humans were exposed to higher levels of simple carbohydrates than their metabolism could handle. As a result, food intolerances, blood glucose imbalance, dyslipidemia, and inflammation threaten public health. Nutrition recommendations for a healthy diet have varied over the years, which creates consumer confusion.

For instance, the goal of dietary counseling during the past 20 years was to achieve and maintain a low-fat diet [6]. Clinical trials of low-fat, high-carbohydrate diets were undertaken to prevent diseases ranging from breast cancer to hyperlipidemia. Yet Dr. Walter Willet of the Harvard School of Public Health told Frontline in 2004.

> There was never any strong evidence for this idea, but it was repeated so often that it became dogma.… This campaign to reduce fat in the diet has had some pretty disastrous consequences.… One of the most unfortunate unintended consequences of the fat-free crusade was the idea that if it wasn't fat, it wouldn't make you fat. I even had colleagues who were telling the public that you can't get fat eating carbohydrates. Actually, farmers have known for thousands of years that you can make animals fat by feeding them grains … and it turns out that applies to human. [7]

Setting Carbohydrate Goals for the Diet

Refined grain diet like white bread, white rice, and white flour comprises approximately, 30% of the calories in the American diet and contains substantially lower amounts of vitamins, minerals, and fiber than unrefined grains [8]. In addition, refined grains are absorbed rapidly and may lead to blood glucose control issues.

Sugar

Nearly 20% of the calories in the typical American diet are derived from added sugars (not including the sugars that occur naturally in fruit, milk, and other unprocessed foods) [8]. This translates into around 40 teaspoons of added sugar per person per day [9] and many bariatric surgery patients consume much more than that. Since refined sugar contains no vitamins, minerals, or micronutrients, added sugar consumption needs to be significantly reduced.

Sweets were once considered a treat but now the average American adult consumes one-third of their calories in sugar and white flour according to Jacob Teitelbaum, MD, in *Complete Guide to Beating Sugar Addiction* [10]. Dr. Teitelbaum outlines four types of sugar addicts, which may be helpful for health-care professionals to keep in mind when designing weight loss management messages pre- and postbariatric surgery.

The type 1 sugar addict is always exhausted and hooked on caffeine and sugar for energy, usually presenting with immune dysfunction. Type 2 is the perpetual crisis person with too much to do and stressed out trying to do everything while juggling blood pressure, blood glucose, and fatigue issues. Type 3 craves sugar to feed the intestinal yeast overgrowth, which causes sinusitis, spastic colon, and food intolerances. Type 4 is depressed with low hormone levels that drive the need for sugar.

Damon Gameau, graphically illustrates what 40 teaspoons of sugar from foods considered beneficial can do to your health in *"That Sugar Film"* [11]. Grace Shearrer et al., at the University of Texas, Austin, studied sugar-sweetened beverage intake and found greater visceral fat in the high-intake group, which was associated with higher cortisol response [12].

Among the world's largest sugar producers in the United States where sugar cane accounts for approximately 45% of the total sugar produced and sugar beets for around 55%, with the United States Department of Agriculture (USDA) production data showing increases over the past three decades [13]. Sugar also plays an important part in food processing and the more processed foods Americans consume, the more sugar they eat.

The best way to reduce sugar intake is to limit consumption of processed foods and drinks, since sugar is an ingredient in three-fourths of all packaged foods and sweetened beverages. Eat, don't drink, your fruits and vegetables and skip bakery products like the bagel (55 g carbohydrate), cinnamon roll (94 g carbohydrate), or cookie (30 g carbohydrate).

Bariatric surgery can curb the sweet tooth by altering the brain's reward system according to a study in *Cell Metabolism* [14]. This study was done in mice and the how and why still need to be worked out in humans. Patients need to start changing food habits before surgery for success by reducing high-calorie, high-sugar foods. Madjd et al. found that the replacement of diet beverages with water led to greater weight reduction and less insulin resistance [15].

Personalizing the carbohydrates in the diet requires assistance in understanding the glycemic index, sugar substitute preferences, and/or dietary fiber recommendations and tolerances. Support groups could focus on these topics to illustrate the importance of these issues.

The concepts of glycemic index and glycemic load are described as a means of classifying carbohydrate foods based on the food's impact on glucose response in the body. A high-glycemic index food is more rapidly converted to glucose [16]. Most breads, breakfast cereals, and grain products have a high glycemic index, whereas most fruits, non-starchy vegetables, and legumes are low glycemic index.

Sugar substitutes (also known as artificial sweeteners or nonnutritive sweeteners or noncaloric sweeteners) are sweeteners that contain virtually no calories and no carbohydrates. They are plant-based or chemical substances that are hundreds of times sweeter than sugar and have no effect on blood glucose levels. Some sugar substitutes can be used in baking to reduce carbohydrate content but flour also contributes to the carbohydrate level in cookies, cakes, and desserts.

Stevia rebaudiana is a plant native to South America and is grown throughout China. *Stevia* was previously sold as a dietary supplement until two companies—Cargill and Merissant—developed an extract that received the Food and Drug Administration generally recognized as safe (FDA GRAS) status in 2008. It is 200–400 times sweeter than sugar [17].

Sucralose is made from sugar by replacing three hydroxyl groups on a sucrose molecule with three chlorine atoms. This process was discovered in 1976, approved for use in food in 1999 and is found in over 5,000 foods and beverages today. Sucralose is 600 times sweeter than sugar [17].

Saccharin, discovered by researchers at Johns Hopkins University in 1878, is the oldest sugar substitute. It was used during sugar shortages in World War I and II and is 300–500 times sweeter than sugar [17]. Monk fruit or swingle fruit (Luo Han Guo) is a native of southern China and is a gourd the size of a lemon. Its extracts, called mogrosides, are 300 times sweeter than sugar and possess antioxidant properties [17].

Acesulfame K (Ace-K) is often combined with other sweeteners and is around 200 times sweeter than sugar. Aspartame sold under the name Equal® or NutraSweet® is around 200 times sweeter than sugar but should not be used by people with phenylketonuria (PKU) disease.

Sugar alcohols are used as sugar replacers in foods—candy, gum, ice cream products. Their sweetness varies because they are not true sugars. Chemically, they are hydrogenated sugars—with an extra hydroxyl group. Erythritol, mannitol, sorbitol, and xylitol are identified on the food label. Sugar alcohols are absorbed more slowly than glucose and are more resistant to digestion but have similar calorie content as sugar. The sugar alcohols that are not digested are fermented in the large intestine that can cause a laxative response [18].

Fiber is a nondigestible carbohydrate that is fermented in the colon and/or excreted in the feces. The fiber that occurs naturally and is intact in foods is called dietary fiber. Nondigestible carbohydrates that are added to foods after being extracted from a natural source or synthesized are called functional fiber [19]. Food manufacturers use fibers as bulking, stabilizing, and thickening agents. Inulin and fructo-oligosaccharide may be used as a fat or sugar replacer or prebiotic [20]. Tolerance to dietary fiber and functional fiber will vary significantly pre- and postsurgery.

Setting Fat Goals for the Diet

Nutrition research suggests that Americans should minimize their consumption of *trans* fatty acids and avoid using polyunsaturated fatty acids for frying and high-temperature cooking so they minimize the formation of potentially toxic lipid peroxides [8, p. 6]. Saturated fats may not be as harmful as commonly believed but high-fat processed foods do not belong in a bariatric surgery patient's diet pre- and postsurgery.

High-fat processed foods have contributed to the accelerated increase in obesity throughout the United States during the past 25 years. New evidence is showing that saturated fat from animal foods—butter, cheese, red meat—may not be the cause of obesity. Hydrogenated vegetable oils are detrimental to human health because they contain *trans* fats, which cause inflammation [21]. They entered the food supply almost a century ago when a chemist reacted liquid vegetable oil with hydrogen to make "substitute butter" called margarine. This processing then produced products like Crisco® (to replace lard) and sticks of margarine (to replace butter). In the 1950s, hydrogenated oils were cheap and shelf stable so cakes, pies, cookies, and crackers could have a shelf life of 3–12 months.

Trans fat can be found in vegetable shortenings, margarines, crackers, cookies, and snack foods, which are fried in partially hydrogenated oils. A small amount of *trans* fat is formed naturally in some animal-based foods [22]. *Trans* fats raise the risk of coronary heart disease. Major food sources of *trans* fats in the American diet [23] are

- 40% cakes, cookies, crackers, pies, bread
- 17% margarine
- 8% fried potatoes
- 5% potato chips, corn chips, popcorn
- 4% household shortening
- 3% salad dressings
- 1% breakfast cereals

The saturated fat and cholesterol myth started in 1913 with a study by Nikolai Anitschkov, MD, on rabbits fed with eggs that caused atherosclerosis. Rabbits are vegetarian and do not have a biochemical mechanism for handling cholesterol in animal foods but it took until 1965 for this research to get discounted [24] and another 40 years for the misconception that animal fats are heart neutral and have no effect on cholesterol/high-density lipoprotein (HDL) ratio or heart disease to become public knowledge [25]. They do provide calories so low-fat animal products need to be chosen for weight reduction.

Animal fats are a mixture of saturated and unsaturated fats according to Professor Fred A. Kummerow. Beef fat is 54% unsaturated, lard is 60% unsaturated, and chicken fat is 70% unsaturated [26]. Therefore, chicken would be easier for bariatric patients to digest postsurgery but lean red meat is not and needs to be avoided. Frank Hu, senior author of a recent study on weight loss, indicated that weight loss diets should be tailored to food preferences with less emphasis on low-fat food choices [27]. Deirde Tobias, ScD, also agrees in a systematic review and meta-analysis of randomized controlled trials that compare various weight loss interventions [28].

Fat contains more than twice the calories per gram of carbohydrates and protein but higher fat diets provide higher satiety and may improve long-term adherence to healthier diet choices. Olive oil and avocados can contribute to a balance of omega 3-6-9 fatty acids in the diet.

Fiber

Dietary fiber is grouped into two categories: water-insoluble and water-soluble. Insoluble fibers—cellulose, lignin, and most hemi-celluloses are found in vegetables, wheat, and other grains. Soluble fibers—pectin, gums, and some hemicelluloses are contained in fruits, oats, barley, and legumes [29].

Fibers have the capacity to hold water and improve transit time through the gut resulting in less constipation and less abdominal straining for the colon that may cause hemorrhoids, varicose veins, and diverticular disease. Soluble fiber combines with liquid in the diet to form a gel that delays emptying time and enhances satiety, which can be helpful in adjustable gastric banding and vertical sleeve gastrectomy. Both soluble and insoluble fiber delays glucose absorption from the small intestine and is useful in diabetes management [8, p. 212].

Adverse effects of dietary fiber usually are related to gastrointestinal symptoms such as abdominal pain. Of particular concern for bariatric patients postsurgery is the use of guar gum (extract of guar bean) products in constipation management that can swell 20 times its original size. Bowel and esophageal obstructions have been reported to the U.S. Food and Drug Administration [30].

Fiber-rich foods like whole grains, fresh fruits, raw vegetables, nuts, and seeds may be consumed prior to surgery but need to be discontinued postsurgery until advised by health-care professionals that it is safe to consume these foods.

An easy way to evaluate fiber content in the diet and review modifications that can help relieve constipation issues postsurgery is as follows:

- Legumes (lentils, beans) 1/2 cup   = 7 g
- Bran cereals 1/2 cup   = 3 g
- Vegetables, raw 1 cup   = 2 g

- Vegetables, cooked 1/2 cup   = 1 g
- Fruit, raw 1 small piece/1/2 banana   = 2 g
- Fruit, canned/frozen 1/2 cup   = 1 g
- Bread, white 1 slice   = 1 g
- Bread, whole grain 1 slice   = 2 g

The dietary intervention of adding soluble fiber from oat bran, pectin, or psyllium is frequently mentioned to bariatric patients struggling with constipation. Other patients may have used these fibers to improve insulin sensitivity and lower lipids. But according to a 2005 article in the *American Journal of Gastroenterology*, only 20% of the patients with slow transit benefited from adding more fiber [31]. For some patients and possibly bariatric surgery patients, adding more fiber could worsen constipation symptoms.

A 2012 meta-analysis [32] reviewed the role of fiber on constipation and determined that it does increase stool frequency but does not improve stool consistency or painful defecation. A review published in the *Cleveland Clinic Journal of Medicine* [33] points out that increasing physical activity is not always helpful.

Since constipation results from other disorders like hypothyroidism and food sensitivities, the primary disorder needs to be treated before evacuation problems are resolved. Dietary changes to increase fiber levels in the diet need to be done over 2–3 weeks according to the Cleveland Clinic study authors. In addition, nutrition supplements—calcium and iron—can cause constipation and may need to be modified to improve bowel function.

Setting Protein Goals in the Diet

Low protein intake may be tolerated by the body for a limited period postsurgery but if it persists, deficiency results causing reduced albumin, decreased muscle mass, and hair loss. Protein malnutrition can occur in bariatric patients and proper food choices are essential to meet amino acid needs.

Dietary proteins provide important biological functions in all human cells and are especially important in bariatric nutrition. Twenty amino acids are the building blocks for proteins and serve as the primary source of nitrogen in the human body. But nitrogen content in various food choices varies greatly. An example of how food choices can influence protein content in the diet is provided in the USDA Agriculture Research Service listing below. The percentage of protein content is provided in selected foods [34] as follows:

- Rice, 7
- Milk, 3
- Cheese, 25
- Asparagus, 2
- Apple, 0
- Tofu, 8
- Beef, 21
- Chicken, 23
- Egg, 13
- Tuna, 26
- Codfish, 18

Protein needs to be eaten throughout the day by bariatric patients in order to insure tissues and body fluids have adequate amino acids. In addition, protein is needed to replace losses throughout the day. Small amounts of intact protein and amino acids are lost in urine and feces when pancreatic enzymes and gut lining cells are sloughed off. The largest quantity of protein loss, in other words, nitrogen loss, results from muscle breakdown and repair.

Protein on the Nutrition Label

The protein analysis for measuring nitrogen content on food labels is performed by either the Kjeldahl or Dumes method. According to Dr. Sam K.C. Chang, Department of Cereal and Food Science, North Dakota State University, the Dumas method is used more frequently in nutrition labeling since it is faster. Both methods include measurement of melamine, a toxic protein adulterant, in the total nitrogen content when declaring protein analysis results [35]. The 2008 Chinese melamine scandal brings this concept into focus. It is called "protein spiking" so that the protein content is inflated. There is no easy way to detect the nitrogen bound proteins from other sources added to protein powders and supplements as adulterants. Free amino acid products are the only way to know the protein levels that are bioavailable [36].

The Nutrition Labeling and Education Act (NLEA) requires percent daily value, which is determined using the Protein Digestibility-Corrected Amino Acid Score (PDCAAS), to be used on the label. Dr. Denise Smith states in *Food Analysis* that time and cost associated with the PDCAAS method, result in the label only expressing the protein amount and not the protein efficiency ratio (PER) [37]. Consequently, using the nutrition label on protein enriched products to assess protein quality and quantity is inaccurate and inadequate for bariatric nutrition needs.

Sarwar and McDonough refute the PER as a better means of protein quality evaluation [38]. They recommend an amino acid score corrected for true digestibility as the most suitable method for predicting protein quality in foods for humans. A detailed method was provided in their analytical chemistry article but no current use of this method has been identified.

Nutritional Quality of Protein

The best method currently available for teaching and evaluation of protein needs for the bariatric patient is the protein quality index, PER designed by the Committee on Amino Acids of the Food and Nutrition Board, National Research Council in 1974 [38]. Each food is rated 0–4 to access quality of amino acid content. The scoring system is easy to understand and no animal or clinical studies are required because the method is determined using the amino acid composition of each food.

- Egg, 3.92
- Fish, 3.55
- Beef, 2.30
- Rice, 2.18
- Peanuts, 1.65
- Wheat, 1.53
- Corn, 1.12
- Lentils, 0.93

The quantity of protein on the nutrition label reflects neither amino acid composition nor digestibility of the protein and can include antinutritional factors that affect the quality according to Denise M. Smith, Department of Food Science and Technology, Ohio State University [39]. Trypsin inhibitors are inactivated by cooking but heat stable antinutrient factors like tannins decrease the nutritional value of proteins. Major sources of tannins outlined in the August 2012 *Culinary Nutrition News* from Clemson University are

- Cereals—barley, sorghum
- Beverages—beer, cider, fruit juices, tea, and red wine
- Chocolate and cocoa powder
- Fruits—apples, berries, grapes, pomegranates
- Legumes—beans, chickpeas, lentils
- Nuts—cashews, peanuts, pecans, walnuts, almonds, pistachios
- Vegetables—squash, rhubarb

Tannins are plant-based polyphenols that are called antioxidants and have been discussed as headache-causing compounds. These compounds affect the nutritional value of foods and beverages because they bind proteins and impair the digestibility of food in animals and humans [40]. Antioxidant benefits of tannin intake may prevent the onset of chronic disease [41] but they interfere with nutrient absorption, which limits their usefulness in a bariatric nutrition regime.

Protein Denaturation

Protein, from the Greek meaning "first" or "foremost," is the most important macronutrient in a bariatric diet. Proteins constitute over half the dry weight of most humans and are the instruments carrying genetic information to the cell [42]. They are large molecules that undergo changes in their structure as they are cleaved into amino acids by digestive enzymes and during the cooking or drying process.

Heat, exposure to extremes in pH, and treatment with certain reagents cause proteins to become insoluble and lose their biological activity without damage to the covalent backbone [43]. This process is known as denaturation or unfolding of their protein structure, which results in a loss of activity when heated to 65°C. A denatured globular protein frequently becomes insoluble in an aqueous solution of pH 7 and usually loses its biological activity. A familiar example of protein denaturation is cooking an egg. The white of the egg or albumen coagulates into a white solid upon heating. It does not revert to a clear solution upon cooling because the heat has changed it or denatured the albumen protein.

Denaturation also explains why most proteins are biologically active over a narrow temperature range 0°C–40°C. Temperatures higher than those, for a living organism can cause hydrogen bond disruption or denaturation [44]. Powdered protein formulas used for sports and bariatric nutrition supplements that are treated with organic solvents and strong acids/bases disrupt the hydrogen bonds leading to denaturation that can thus fail to meet bariatric patients' protein needs.

Bioavailability

Protein bioavailability relates to how much protein the body absorbs and can potentially be used for normal healthy body function. Many protein product formulations are based on taste and convenience over bioavailability. That may serve the athletic/sports market but not the bariatric nutrition user.

Food and dietary supplements need to provide only what the body can absorb. Protein supplements are probably the most popular sports nutrition product on the market because of the interest in muscle building with proteins derived from a range of sources—whey, soy, hemp, pea, and algae. Bariatric patients are increasingly using the heavily marketed sports nutrition products for their source of high-protein supplements because of their lower cost and convenient availability.

Free Amino Acids versus Protein Powders

Amino acids are required for every function in the human body. Nine of the twenty amino acids required for synthesis of proteins cannot be produced in human tissues and must be provided by the diet. In addition, individual amino acids play an important part in producing hormones and neurotransmitters, detoxification of chemicals, and antioxidant protection along with bile acid production for digestion [45].

The need and pool of amino acids is so important for metabolism that therapeutic supplementation needs to be considered for each bariatric surgery patient because food proteins are slow to be digested and absorbed into the blood while amino acid needs are continually required for all tissues—gut, muscles, and brain.

Free amino acids are pure and have rapid uptake in the blood so they are available to reduce fatigue, promote DNA and RNA synthesis, and hormone production [46, p. 178]. Estimates of average protein intake required to sustain amino acid status are of VERY limited usefulness [46, p. 180]. Amino acid testing, which may be helpful for patients with chronic fatigue, depression, and bipolar disorders, is available. L-tryptophan is needed in every human tissue for rebuilding every cell yet many bariatric patients come into nutrition counseling on selective serotonin reuptake inhibitors (SSRI) drugs which deplete tryptophan. Without free amino acid supplementation, the dietary tryptophan needed for serotonin synthesis will not be met, resulting in mood, sleep, appetite, and neuropsychiatric disorders like depression, migraine, and anxiety [46, p. 183].

Bariatric nutrition protein supplements that are currently available on the market have insufficient research about the amino acid bioavailability of the protein sources and composition. Of particular concern is digestibility when lactose-containing products predominate the market.

Protein supplements made from whey—the waste product of the dairy industry's cheese manufacturing—is exposed to acid processing and high drying temperatures that reduce bioavailability. In addition, the *Journal of Food Science* in October 2015 reported a study regarding the bleaching methods of whey protein isolates affecting functionality. Most of the fluid whey produced in the United States is derived from cheddar cheese curds with annatto coloring and needs to be bleached to remove the yellow color. The soluble protein level is decreased and protein degradation occurs [47].

As Stephan van Vliet et al. state in the *Journal of Nutrition*, efficacy of dietary strategies on muscle protein synthesis remains to be studied. The use of plant-based proteins versus animal-based proteins needs further evaluation. Grass-fed bovine milk and animal amino acids need to be compared with plant-based proteins with or without leucine supplementation [48]. A high whey protein, leucine and vitamin D_3 enriched supplement was used to reduce the risk of sarcopenia [49]. Bojsen-Moller et al. reported that post Roux-en-Y gastric bypass (RYGB) basal plasma leucine concentrations did not change but caseinate digestion and amino acid absorption accelerated, resulting in faster and higher plasma amino acids [50]. The need for selected amino acid supplementation in bariatric formulas requires further research for improved patient health and well-being.

Bariatric surgery modifies the gastrointestinal tract, changing the pepsin and hydrochloric acid available for protein digestion. Reducing the stomach size changes the level of positively charged hydrogen (stomach acid) produced by parietal cells. These cells begin the digestion of protein ingested and activate pepsin, the main gastric enzyme produced by stomach cells. Without the intrinsic factor produced by parietal cells, transport of vitamin B_{12} to the ileum is compromised. Digestive enzymes may be needed by individuals unable to achieve healthy plasma albumin and protein levels.

Quality of Protein Products

Consumer Reports magazine in 2010 reported on 15 protein powders and drinks purchased in the New York metropolitan area or online for testing levels of arsenic, cadmium, lead, and mercury [51]. Three products were found to contain heavy metals exceeding United States Pharmacopeia (USP) limits. Three daily servings of ready-to-drink liquid EAS Myoplex Original Rich Dark Chocolate Shake, Muscle Milk Chocolate powder, and Muscle Milk Vanilla Creme exceeded lead and arsenic levels while Muscle Milk Nutritional Shake Chocolate liquid approached the USP limit.

Cadmium levels were of special concern since it accumulates in the body and can lead to kidney damage. Food sources like shellfish and liver can be high in cadmium, along with potatoes, rice, and sunflower seeds, which take up the metal from cadmium-containing fertilizers, but these foods are not consumed three times a day for months at a time like bariatric surgery patients need to do after surgery.

Robert Wright, MD, associate professor at Harvard Medical School who studies the health effects of toxic metal exposure indicates that exposure to small amounts is inevitable but products that exceed

USP limits are not recommended [51]. When products with this toxic mixture are regularly consumed, they target the same organs and have a synergistic effect making two toxic substances greater than the sum of the two. Not enough research has been done to fully understand long terms effects of protein powders and drinks that contain toxic metals, according to Dr. Wright.

The web-based Labdoor testing results of high-protein products identified label inaccuracies and inactive ingredients found in the 74 products analyzed. "Over 52% of the products analyzed had measurable amounts of free-form amino acids, which spike protein content in standard laboratory tests but add little nutritional benefit," according to the website [52].

Two food testing laboratories were contacted for an independent analysis of several products reported as being used by patients. Each declined the request to provide an analysis of the products stating that it was a "conflict of interest" since they produce the nutrition labels for companies sending their products to them for evaluation.

Protein powders made from a low-heat, nonchemical extraction process, free of gluten and lectins with no artificial colors and flavors would have efficient utilization in the body for bariatric surgery patients. Using amino acid powders and/or free amino capsules is another cost-effective way to ensure that high biological value protein is available in the bariatric diet. Little attention has been paid to individual differences in amino acid requirements to maintain nitrogen equilibrium [53], and the Recommended Dietary Allowances (RDAs) that were developed by the Food and Nutrition Board of the Research Council do not address biochemical needs of individuals, so relevancy of the nutrition label to evaluate products for bariatric patients is fraudulent.

Clinical Issues in Protein Nutrition

As Arne Astrup's editorial in the *American Journal of Clinical Nutrition* points out, protein increases satiety even if the effect is not explained by changes in the hunger hormone ghrelin or the satiety hormone leptin [54]. The high-protein diets of Atkins, the Zone, and the South Beach Diet seem to point in the direction of increasing protein recommendations by 30%–40% of the calorie content, at the expense of carbohydrates. The protein needs for bariatric surgery patients should have top priority in research with adequate testing done by laboratories specializing in amino acid profiles.

Dietary protein needs for a moderately fasting bariatric surgery patient are currently calculated as 1.2–1.4 g protein per kg ideal body weight based on approximately, 250 g protein turnover in a day for the average adult [38, p. 46]. Muscle protein turnover equals approximately, 65 g/day or around one-fourth of the total turnover according to Shills et al. A 300 lb. bariatric patient whose ideal body weight or weight loss goal is 180 lb. would need 98 g (82 kg × 1.2 g) to 115 g (82 kg × 1.4 g) protein daily. Faria et al. conclude that care should be taken to ensure that bariatric patients consume not only high-quality protein supplements (60–120 g/day) but that it includes good quality proteins like meat, eggs, and cheese [55]. An example of meal plan to provide adequate amino acids, based on USDA database analysis, follows [56]. It emphasizes the importance of small frequent meals and high-quality protein at each snack/meal for use during the first months postsurgery.

8 AM   smoothie: 4 scoops amino acid powder* + 1/4 cup plain yogurt, 1/2 banana, 1/2 cup mixed berries, 1/2 cup water

10 AM   2 oz. yogurt with 1 scoop amino acid powder*

Noon   2 oz. cottage Cheese and pureed peaches

2 PM   2 oz. tuna fish salad + 1 scoop amino acid powder* mixed in

4 PM   smoothie with 4 scoops amino acid powder* + 1/2 banana, 1/2 tablespoon cocoa powder, 1/4 cup plain yogurt, 1/2 cup water

6 PM   2 oz. cream cheese or goat cheese with 1 scoop amino acid powder,* one small baked potato or 1/4 cup mashed potato

8 PM   1/2 cup ice cream or fruit ice with 1 scoop amino acid powder*

---

* Pure Encapsulations Amino Replete (2 scoops/4 teaspoons = 1/4 cup cottage cheese or 1 egg)

Cold-processed whey protein concentrate is an alternative to amino acid capsules or powder. Whey protein isolate products are not recommended because they are stripped of nutrition cofactors in the production of the powder and primarily provide only calories.

Look for labels that read "free of genetically modified organisms (GMO) ingredients," pesticides and chemicals. Cows fed GMO corn and soy have glyphosphates in the milk and whey. The World Health Organization has indicated glyphosphate is a probable carcinogen.

References

1. Kusher R, Still CD, eds. *Nutrition and Bariatric Surgery*. Boca Raton, FL: CRC Press, 2015.
2. Dor A, Ferguson C, Langwith CL, et al. A heavy burden: The individual costs of being overweight and obese in the United States. Washington, DC: Department of Health Policy, School of Public Health and Health Services, George Washington University, 2010.
3. Vesely JM, De Mattia LG. Obesity: Dietary and lifestyle management. *Family Physician Essent* 2014 Oct;425:11–15.
4. Parker K, O'Brien P, Brennan L. Measurement of disordered eating following bariatric surgery: A systematic review of the literature. *Obes Surg* 2014;24:945–953.
5. Trust for America's Health and the Robert Wood Johnson Foundation. The State of Obesity. 2015. Available at: http://stateofobesity.org.
6. White E, Shattuck AL, Kristal AR, et al. Maintenance of a low fat diet: Follow-up of the women's health trial. *Cancer Epidemiol Biomarkers Prev* 1992 May–Jun; 1(4):315–323.
7. Willet W. Did the low-fat era make us fat? [Online interview] Frontline. www.pbs.org/wgbh/pages/frontline/shows/diet/themes/lowfat.html.
8. Gaby AJ. *Nutritional Medicine*. Concord, NH: Fritz Perlberg publishing, 2011, p. 5.
9. Elliott SS, Keim NL, Stern JS, et al. Fructose, weight gain and the insulin resistance syndrome. *Am J Clin Nutr* 2002;76:911–922.
10. Teitelbaum J, Fiedler C. *The Complete Guide to Beating Sugar Addiction*. Beverly, MA: Fair Winds Press, 2015.
11. O'Connor A. A spoonful of medicine about sugar. *New York Times*, Aug 18, 2015.
12. Shearrer GE et al. The relationship between sugar-sweetened beverage intake, cortisol response and fat partitioning. *Endocrine Today*. Dec 2015.
13. Mermelstein NH. More than a spoonful of sugar. *Food Technology* 2015 Nov;67–69.
14. Han W, Tellez LA, Niu J, et al. Striatal dopamine links gastrointestinal rerouting to altered sweet appetite. *Cell Metabolism* 2016 Oct;23:103–112.

15. Madjd A, Taylor MA, Delavari A, et al. Effects on weight loss in adults of replacing diet beverages with water during a hypoenergetic diet: A randomized, 24-week clinical trial. *Am J Clin Nutr* 2015;102:1305–1312.

16. Bell S, Sears B. Low glycemic-load diets: Impact on obesity and chronic diseases. *Crit Rev Food Sci Nutr* 2003;43(4):357–377.

17. Campbell A. Baking and cooking with sugar substitutes. *Diabetes Self Management.* 2015 Oct;32(5):18–21.

18. Grabitske HA, Slavin JL. Low digestible carbohydrates in practice. *J Amer Diet Assoc* 2008 Oct;108(10):1677–1687.

19. Institute of Medicine. *Dietary Reference Intakes: Proposed Definitions of Dietary Fiber.* Food and nutrition board National Academy of Sciences Washington, DC: National Academy Press, 2001.

20. Roberfroid MB. Inulin-type fructans: Functional food ingredients. *J Nutr* 2007;137(11):S2493–2502.

21. Johnson PV, Johnson OC, Kummerow FA. Occurrence of trans fatty acids in human tissue. *Science* 1957;126:698–699.

22. What Is Trans Fat? *FDA Consumer Magazine.* Sept–Oct 2003 Issue Pub No FDA 05-1329C, revised Sept. 2005.

23. USDA Composition data from What Is Trans Fat? *FDA Consumer Magazine.* Sept—Oct 2003 Issue Pub No FDA 05-1329C, revised Sept. 2005.

24. Kritchevsky D, Tepper SA. Factors affecting atherosclerosis in rabbits fed cholesterol-free diets. *Life Sci* 1965;4:1467–1471.

25. Pinckney ER, Smith RL. Statistical analysis of lipid research clinics program. *Lancet* 1987;1(8531):503–504.

26. Passwater RA. From pellagra to trans fats and beyond—How a legendary nutritional scientist is still saving countless thousands from premature deaths. *Whole Foods Magazine.* 2014 Oct;37(10):48–52.

27. Hu FB, Tobias DK, Chen M et al . Low fat diet not most effective in long term weight loss. *Lancet Diabetes Endocrinology* 2015 Oct; 3(12):915–1016.

28. Tobias DK. Chen M, Manson JE, et al. Effect of low-fat diet interventions versus other diet interventions on long-term weight change in adults: A systematic review and meta-analysis. Lancet *Diabetes Endocrinol* 2015 Oct; 3(12):968–979.

29. Anderson JW. Fiber and health: An overview. *Am J Gastroenterol* 1986;81:892–897.

30. Lewis JH. Esophageal and small bowel obstruction from guar gum-containing "diet pills": Analysis of 26 cases reported to the Food and Drug Association. *Am J Gastroenterol* 1992;87:1424–1428.

31. Muller-Lissner SA, Kamm MA, et al. Myths and misconceptions about chronic constipation. *Am J Gastroenterol* 2005;100(1):232–242.

32. Yang J, Wang HP, Zhou L, et al. Effect of dietary fiber on constipation: A meta-analysis. *World J Gastroenterol* 2012;18(48): 7378–7383.

33. Foxx-Orenstein AE, McNally MA, et al. Update on constipation: One treatment does not fit all. *Cleve Clin J Med* 2008;75(11):813–824.

34. USDA, ARS. www.ars.usda.gov/bhnrc/ndl.

35. Chang SKC. In: SS Nielsen (ed.) *Food Analysis*, New York, NY: Springer, 2010.

36. Lovett RA. Six more dietary ingredients picked for analytical evaluation. *Nutraceutical World*. March 2016.

37. Smith DM. In: SS Nielsen (ed.) *Food Analysis*. New York, NY: Springer 2010.

38. Sarwar G, McDonough FE. Evaluation of protein digestibility-corrected amino acid score method for assessing protein quality of foods. *J Assoc of Anal Chem* 1990;May–June;73(3);347–356.

39. Shills ME, Shike M, Ross AC, et al. *Modern Nutrition in Health and Disease*, Tenth Edition. Baltimore, MD: Lippincott Williams and Wilkins, 2006, pp. 55–56.

40. Culinary Nutrition Articles: Lingering Tannins. *Culinary Nutrition News*, Clemson University. Available at: www.clemson.edu.

41. Serrano J, Puupponen-Pimia R, Dauer A, et al. Tannins: Current knowledge of food sources, intake, bioavailability and biological effects. *Mol Nutr Food Res* 2009;53 (Suppl 2):S310–329.

42. Lila MA. From beans to berries and beyond: Teamwork between plant chemicals for protection of optimal human health. *Ann NY Acad Sci.* 2007;1114:372–380.

43. Nelson DL, Cox MM. *Lehninger Principles of Biochemistry*, Sixth Edition. New York, NY: Macmillan, 2012.

44. Champe PC, Harvey RA, Ferrier DR. *Biochemistry*, Third Edition. Philadelphia, PA: Lippincott Williams and Wilkins, 2005, p. 470.

45. Seager S, Slabaugh MR. *Organic and Biochemistry for Today*, Sixth Edition. Boston, MA: Thomson Learning, 2008.

46. Lord RS, Bralley JA. *Laboratory Evaluations for Integrative and Functional Medicine*, Second Edition. Duluth, GA: Metametrix Institute, 2008, p. 178.

47. Smith TJ, Foegeding EA, Drake M. Sensory and functionality difference in whey protein isolate bleached by hydrogen or benzoyl peroxide. *J of Food Science* 2015 Oct;80(10):2153–2160.

48. van Vliet S, Burd NA, van Loon LJ. The skeletal muscle anabolic response to plant- verus animal-based protein consumption. *J Nut* 2015;145:1981–1991.

49. Verreijen AM, Verlaan S, Engberink MF et al. A high whey protein-, leucine-, and vitamin D-enriched supplement preserves muscle mass during intentional weight loss in obese older adults: A double-blind randomized controlled trial. *Am J Clin Nutr* 2015;101:279–286.

50. Bojsen-Moller KN, Jacobsen SH, Dirksen C, et al. Accelerated protein digestion and amino acid absorption after Roux-en-Y gastric bypass. *Am J Clin Nutr* 2015;102:600–607.

51. *Consumer Reports Magazine*, July 2010.

52. Labdoor.com https://labdoor.com

53. Williams RJ. *Individuality in nutrition. Biochemical Individuality.* New Canaan, CT: Keats Publishing, 1998.

54. Astrup A. The satiety power of protein-a key to obesity prevention. *Am J Clin Nutr* 2005;82:1–2.
55. Faria SL, Faria OP, Buffington C, et al. Dietary protein intake and bariatric surgery patients: A review. *Obes Surg* 2011;21:1798–1805.
56. USDA Database for Standard Reference 2002.

6

DIETARY SUPPLEMENTS— PRE- AND POSTSURGERY

Bariatric surgery is associated with lifelong nutritional deficiencies, which can have deleterious effects on health and well-being. The malabsorptive procedures produced by the surgery is associated with deficiencies in B vitamins and fat-soluble vitamins A, D, E, and K along with the minerals—zinc, magnesium, iron, and copper. There is a great variability in the recommendation of dietary supplements despite the significant effects on the surgical outcome and weight loss success.

With more than two-thirds of American adults taking dietary supplements, there are a number of responsible manufacturers who provide safe products. Because consumers are constantly bombarded with information they need to consider product comparisons for quality and quantity pre- and postbariatric surgery. They cannot afford to pay for dietary supplements that do not provide a high return on their investment.

Ensuring production of pharmaceutical grade dietary supplements with a Good Manufacturing Practice (GMP) designation on the label is the best way to start the evaluation process for safety and efficacy. Supplement providers need to be able to provide a Certificate of Analysis (COA) on their products to verify high-quality ingredients analyzed by a laboratory independent of their facility for pureness and bioavailability. In the absence of that level of verification, consumers should look elsewhere for dietary supplements. Over 50% of supplement users consider their health-care professionals as a trusted source for reliable information, so clinics should verify any/all products they provide to patients.

Some bariatric surgery patients have even purchased weight loss products via the Internet only to realize that the Federal Trade Commission (FTC) and U.S. Department of Justice have filed a suit against the company for manufacturing dietary supplements under conditions that do not meet U.S. Food and Drug Administration's current GMP requirements [1]. Careful vetting of products recommended to patients is necessary.

Unfortunately, health-care professionals understand the benefits of dietary supplements but lack evidence-based research because such studies are expensive. To improve the quality of life for bariatric surgery patients, unhealthy behaviors need to be changed and healthier nutrition choices in food and supplements need to be implemented.

Until insurers provide full coverage for dietary supplements for bariatric patients, health-care providers need to recommend products to meet the individual health needs of each patient and emphasize that cost should not be the only factor in selecting a supplement pre- and postsurgery.

Need for Dietary Supplements

Food is a source of nutrients for the human body, despite how it is grown or prepared. Macro- and micronutrient deficiencies are frequently an issue in obese individuals who have been choosing high-calorie, low-quality foods because of price, taste, or convenience.

Presurgery supplementation can reduce mortality rates [2] and allow for better nutrition habits for supplementation to be established. Preoperative nutrient deficiencies have been reported for vitamin D, ferritin, hemoglobin, vitamin B_{12}, and thiamine [3]. Nutrition guidelines should include at least one excellent multivitamin and mineral capsule daily. Postsurgery this supplement capsule can then be opened up and added to beverages and soft foods.

Postsurgery patients consume a liquid diet for the first week, which needs to provide liquid dietary supplements to maintain muscle mass and improve immune function [4]. By week two they can usually progress to capsule supplements that can be opened and incorporated into liquids. Crushing of tablets is not recommended because absorption is significantly impaired [5].

Bioavailability

The debate about bioavailability of dietary supplements focuses on absorption. Since dietary supplements are NOT pharmaceuticals, there is no requirement to access for disintegration. Tablets are made by mixing ingredients and compressing them with additives to form a specified size and shape. Tablets are lower in cost, offered in elegant sizes and shapes, and may have enteric coatings to reduce gastrointestinal irritation. But the excessive compaction from pressure processing leads to poor bioavailability and many pass intact into the feces.

Capsules usually have vegetable source shells that protect the nutrients from acidification in the stomach. They are easier to swallow with reduced gastrointestinal distress but capsules are more difficult to fill, which increases cost.

Gummy supplements may lead the way in taste and acceptance but any nutrient in them is exposed to the harsh stomach environment for denaturation and the gooeyness on the teeth can promote dental issues.

The Association of Official Agricultural Chemists (AOAC) is continuing to help the dietary supplement industry agree on and evaluate analytical methods to ensure quality, safety, and regulatory compliance. Twenty-five "priority ingredients" have been chosen to be evaluated by the 131-year-old AOAC organization under a contract funded by the National Institute of Health (NIH), Office of Dietary Supplements [6]. More information is available on the AOAC website: www.AOAC.org.

Postoperative Nutrition Monitoring

Monitoring of the food choices and nutrition supplement use is needed, especially postoperatively, for ensuring weight loss and identification of nutrient deficiencies. The medical literature suggests that several key nutrients need to be assessed after surgery—vitamin B_{12}, folate, vitamin D, vitamin K, selenium, zinc, and copper [3].

Vitamin B_{12}

Vitamin B_{12} is a group of cobalt containing compounds described by Alan R. Gaby, MD, in *Nutritional Medicine* called cobalamins.

Methylcobalamin is the coenzyme form of B_{12} that is critical for human health. Hydroxocobalamin is a more stable form of B_{12} but it first needs to be converted to an active form before it can be used in metabolism [7, pp. 89–96]. The most inexpensive form of vitamin B_{12} is cyanocobalamin, containing cyanide and found in most multivitamin formulas because of its cost effectiveness.

Vitamin B_{12} is important in DNA synthesis, red blood cell (RBC) formation, homocysteine (HCY) metabolism, and the production of S-adenosylmethionine (SAMe). Adequate B_{12} is essential for proper neurological and immune functioning.

The importance of vitamin B_{12} in health and anemia management was first realized during the Depression era when animal protein foods were limited in the American diet. Three physicians who reversed pernicious anemia in dogs were awarded the 1934 Nobel Prize for medicine. Drs. George Hoyt Whipple, George Richards Minot, and William Parry Murphy fed the dogs and humans 1/2 lb. of fresh liver per day as a means to control anemia [8].

Animal proteins—meat, poultry, fish, eggs—are the sources of vitamin B_{12} for humans. Plants do not need or produce B_{12}. How B_{12} gets into your blood is a complex dance of stomach acids and intrinsic factors that starts with pepsin in the stomach splitting off the B_{12} from the protein compound to which it is bound. The intrinsic factor made by the parietal cells of the stomach attaches to the B_{12} to be shuttled to the ileum where receptors pull it into the blood [9]. Once in the blood, B_{12} is picked up by transcobalamin to be carried to cells throughout the body. Any excess is stored in the liver or excreted in the urine.

If inadequate intrinsic factor is available—loss from aging or proton pump inhibitor (PPI) use—B_{12} deficiency symptoms such as macrocytic anemia, neurological disorders, and psychiatric symptoms (memory loss, depression, confusion, paranoia) may occur. Severe B_{12} deficiency can result in intestinal damage, hyperpigmentation of the skin, hypotension, and immune dysfunction.

The Institute of Medicine (IOM) indicates that only 2–4 µg vitamin B_{12} is needed daily. The average American diet contains 5–15 µg per day according to the National Health and Nutrition Examination Survey (NHANES) studies [10]. Vegetarians and infants breastfed by vegan mothers are at greatest risk of developing B_{12} deficiency [11].

Despite the adequacy of IOM and NHANES data, other factors increase the risk of developing vitamin B_{12} insufficiency. Achlorhydria secondary to gastritis, gastric bypass surgery, and ileal resection for Crohn's disease need assessment due to malabsorption [12]. Apathy abounds throughout the medical community despite the 2009 Centers for Disease Control and Prevention statistics indicating 1 out of every 31 persons over 50 years being B_{12} deficient [13]. With increasing numbers of gastric bypass patients, this deficiency could be significantly higher.

Adverse symptoms can first be noted with the complete blood count (CBC) test indicating large RBCs or macrocytosis—a folate and B_{12} deficiency. Other symptoms may include balance problems, numb hands and feet, leg pains, early onset dementia, pre-Parkinson's-like disease, infertility, and depression.

Many physicians are poorly educated on vitamin B_{12} importance since it is a vitamin and easy to treat. Treatment with methylcobalamin injections with few definitive ways to test efficacy seems to be a primary factor. A complete medical history assessing for gut inflammation, celiac disease, gastroesophageal reflux disease (GERD), recent nitric oxide use in surgery, and genetic factors like methylene tetrahydrofolate reductase (MTHFR) should trigger a closer look at B_{12} adequacy even with a normal HCY plasma test [14]. According to Lewerin et al. high levels of B_{12} on standard blood analysis usually indicates poor absorption not intoxification of vitamin B_{12}. Elevated B_{12} results >800 pg/mL frequently can indicate PPI use, low-stomach acid, or malabsorption. B_{12} lab results <350 pg/mL may still be inadequate for a patient with celiac disease, gluten enteropathy, or gastric bypass surgery so supplementation should be considered.

Medications matter when considering vitamin B_{12} status. Following are common drugs that impair absorption [8, pp. 30–31]:

- Antacids—maalox, milk of magnesia (MOM), Mylanta, Tums
- Histamine blockers—Zantac, Tagamet, Axid, Pepcid
- PPIs—Prevacid, Prilosec, Nexium, Omeprazole, Aciphex
- Colchicine
- Questran
- Metformin, Glucophage
- Celexa, Effexor, Elavil, Nardil, Paxil, Prozac, Zoloft, Wellbutrin
- Ativan, Librium, Valium, Xanax

- Viagra, Cialis, Levitra
- Compazine, Haldol, Risperdal, Tegretal

Vitamin B_{12} supplementation is probably the safest medical treatment available and many bariatric patients may need B_{12} injections to show improvement in their symptoms. Effectiveness of injections depends more on frequency of administration than on amount given with each injection. Those who improve with injections rarely improve with oral or sublingual products no matter how large the dose because oral routes of administration are not capable of achieving high enough absorption levels [15].

Treatment with vitamin B_{12} may need to be continued for life. Until more research on efficacy and safety of oral B_{12} is available, intramuscular daily or weekly injections should be considered a standard of care, especially for those with gastric bypass surgery. Supplementation effectiveness can improve patient outcome as reviewed by Moore and Sherman [16].

Vitamin B_{12} is primarily found in animal protein foods—egg yolks, meat, fish, and yogurt with grass-fed beef liver as an excellent source. Tempeh, a fermented soybean product, and some sprouts may contain in modest amounts. Vitamin B_{12} in food is easily destroyed by microwave cooking.

Folate (Folic Acid)

Folic acid is the synthetic form of folate used in dietary supplements and food fortification. It needs to be converted into biologically active folate to be available in the synthesis of DNA and RNA [7]. Folate is also critical in HCY and vitamin B_{12} metabolism. Folate is essential in cardiovascular, dermatological, neurological, and psychological conditions ranging from atherosclerosis, psoriasis, migraine headaches to depression.

Absorption of folic acid/folate requires gastric hydrochloric acid [17] with bioavailability of folic acid supplements approximately, 100% when assessed in healthy volunteers [18] but the folate present in food is only one-third to one-half bioavailable [19]. Individuals with MTHFR genetic factors are encouraged to select methylfolate products (also called Optimized Folate, FolaPro or 5-MTHFR).

The supplement label must read folate NOT folic acid. Higher dose prescription products—Deplin and Metanx—are available especially for those taking high dose niacin or for treating depression.

The supplement label must read L-form of folate, not the D-form, an example: L-methyltetrahydrofolate. The U.S. Food and Drug Administration is proposing a rule on vitamin labels that only folic acid can be used on supplements because folate is found in foods. Hopefully this designation will not be forthcoming due to the confusion it would cause.

Megaloblastic anemia is the best recognized sign of folate deficiency. Other symptoms usually associated with insufficiency are depression, anxiety, fatigue, apathy, confusion, and dementia [20]. Severe folate deficiency may cause neurological disorders similar to those in vitamin B_{12} deficiency. Low folate can also lead to malabsorption of other nutrients, which can be of concern in bariatric surgery patients [21].

The absence of macrocytic anemia should not rule out folate deficiency. Serum folate laboratory testing fluctuates according to dietary intake. The RBC folate levels are the more stable form to access but may be influenced by vitamin B_{12} deficiency and/or iron deficiency.

Food sources of folate include leafy green vegetables, legumes, and citrus fruits. Foods highly processed or overcooked have reduced availability of folate. For increased bioavailability, raw or lightly steamed vegetables need to be consumed because the conjugase enzymes in the vegetables cause inactivation of the folates from heat [22].

B Complex Vitamins

Vitamin B complex includes a group of eight vitamins.

Thiamin is a vital part of coenzyme thiamine pyrophosphate for energy metabolism. Major food sources include whole grains and pork [23].

Riboflavin serves as a coenzyme in many reactions for energy metabolism. Food sources include liver, eggs, and dairy products [23].

Niacin, also known as niacinamide, participates in numerous metabolic actions, especially glucose, fat, and alcohol metabolism. Food sources include meat, chicken, tuna, and liver [23].

Biotin is critical as a coenzyme for gluconeogenesis and fatty acid synthesis. Food sources include egg yolk, fish, and whole grains [23].

Pantothenic acid is a B vitamin with involvement in more than 100 metabolic pathways such as lipid metabolism and neurotransmitter, hemoglobin, and hormone functions. Food sources include beef, whole grains, tomatoes, broccoli, and avocado [23].

Vitamin B_6 occurs in three forms—pyridoxal, pyridoxine, and pyridoxamine—which is needed for amino acid metabolism. Deficiency causes neurotransmitter issues that include depression, confusion, and abnormal brain wave patterns. It is easily destroyed by heat with primary food sources being meat, fish, poultry, legumes, and liver [23].

Due to limited consumption from bariatric surgery, patients may need to consider supplementation.

Vitamin C

Vitamin C serves as a cofactor in enzyme function and as an antioxidant. It protects tissues from oxidative stress and plays an important role in preventing chronic diseases. Vitamin C helps form the fibrous connective tissues known as collagen for bone and teeth formation. The food sources include broccoli, strawberries, kiwi, and bell peppers [23].

Due to limited consumption from bariatric surgery, patients may need to consider supplementation.

Vitamin D

Vitamin D is a fat-soluble prohormone synthesized by the skin when it is exposed to ultraviolet B (UVB) radiation. Vitamin D comes in two forms—D_2 (ergocalciferol) and D_3 (cholecalciferol). Vitamin D_2 is synthesized for use in dietary supplements and fortified foods. Vitamin D_3 is synthesized as a result of skin exposure to the sun and also occurs naturally in some animal foods—egg yolks, fatty fish, cod liver oil [7, pp. 108–111].

Medicine has regarded these two vitamers of vitamin D as equivalent and interchangeable according to the *American Journal of Clinical Nutrition* but this conclusion is outdated and bariatric health professionals need to reconsider their recommendations accordingly [7, pp. 108–111]. Previously, vitamins D, D_2, and D_3 were considered equivalent based on studies that evaluated their ability to prevent rickets in children. Today, vitamin D status needs to be assessed on calcidiol or 25-hydroxyvitamin D metabolite activity. According to the comparative study of vitamin D_2 and vitamin D_3 supplementation, vitamin D_3 was considered more potent and less toxic at higher doses than vitamin D_2.

Both D_2 and D_3 are biologically inert until they undergo two hydroxylation reactions. The first is in the liver to form 25-hydroxyvitamin D (25[OH]D). It is then further hydroxylated in the kidney to 1,25-dihydroxyvitamin D (1,25[OH]2 D) [7, pp. 108–111].

Vitamin D promotes bone mineralization, neurological and immune function, and influences cell growth and repair. Occurrence of malabsorption in chronic liver disease, pancreatic insufficiency, celiac/gluten sensitivity, and Crohn's disease has been reported [24]. Evaluation of vitamin D levels in bariatric patients needs to be done to assess prevalence and need.

Deficiency symptoms in adults present as bone pain, muscle weakness, and fatigue. Individuals, who have limited sun exposure and rely on vitamin D_2 supplementation, may not achieve desirable serum levels because of reduced stability and bioavailability of D2 [25].

Adiposity also impacts vitamin D status. People with larger amounts of adipose tissue increase their calcidiol levels only half as much as people with lower fat mass when given similar doses of vitamin D. Adipocytes sequester vitamin D and the relevance of this relationship needs further exploration [26].

To reach a healthy calcidiol level, the IOM recommends a daily vitamin D intake of 600 IU until age 70, then 800 IU for older Americans. The optimal dose of vitamin D remains a research question. A number of studies indicate 800 IU/day provides better benefit than 400 IU/day. Some studies have found that 25(OH)D can be increased with daily, weekly, or monthly supplementation—1,500 IU/day or 10,500 IU weekly or 45,000 IU monthly [27]. Other studies recommend daily supplementation to be more effective [28].

Moderate sunshine exposure may be the best method to obtain vitamin D with the exposure of arms, legs, and face 5–15 minutes, two to three times daily between 10 AM and 3 PM, April to October [29]. As Chan et al. indicate, vitamin D status postbariatric surgery is critical for assessment and repletion [30].

Food sources of vitamin D_3 are fish liver oil (cod liver oil), egg yolks, butter, and grass-fed beef liver. Homogenized milk and most cereals are "fortified" with synthetic vitamin D.

Vitamin K

Vitamin K is a general term used to describe several related compounds. vitamin K_1 or phylloquinone is the form found in plants—predominately leafy greens and vegetable oils. Vitamin K_2 is referred to as menaquinone and is found in animal foods—egg yolks, meats, cheese curds, and fermented foods like natto (fermented soybeans) [31].

Vitamin K deficiency can lead to major bleeding problems since green vegetables, salads, and fat sources are significantly reduced in the bariatric diet. Vitamin K_2 loss may result in bone loss or osteoporosis [32].

Vitamin K_1 deficiency can be identified by an elevated International Normalization Ratio (INR) or prothrombin time. Although deficiency is seldom severe enough to cause bleeding, lack of adequate food intake in conditions like inflammatory bowel disease and celiac/gluten sensitivity have been reported to lead to malabsorption [33]. The bariatric diet results in low intake, which may contribute to malabsorption issues.

Selenium

Selenium functions as a cofactor for glutathione peroxidase for detoxification and immune enhancement in addition to treatment of congestive heart failure, hepatitis, lymphedema, thyroiditis, and cancer [7, pp. 166–168]. The selenium content of foods depends on the selenium content of the soil where it is grown. Vegetarians have significantly lower selenium status than omnivores probably related to protein quality and methionine levels in their food choices [34].

Alasfar et al. report selenium status needs review presurgery [35]. Food sources of selenium include meat, fish, legumes, and Brazil nuts but since consumption is limited by bariatric surgery, supplementation beyond multivitamins and minerals may be needed for those with thyroid disorders.

Zinc

Zinc is an important cofactor in numerous biochemical pathways including DNA and protein synthesis. It is essential for growth and functions as an antioxidant for cell membrane stabilization [7, pp. 151–157].

Absorption of zinc is dependent on age and content in the diet [36]. Deficiency is related to impaired taste sensation, anorexia, impaired mental awareness, diarrhea, low testosterone, anemia, impaired wound healing, and alopecia [37]. Because of the lack of laboratory testing to identify zinc deficiency, clinical assessment could include presence of white spots on the fingernails [38] and signs of immune dysfunction like frequent infections.

Supplementation using zinc sulfate 220 mg three times a day (equivalent to 50 mg elemental zinc) has been shown to be less bioavailable and not well tolerated. Other preparations like zinc citrate and picolinate are better tolerated.

Food sources include seafood, meats, wheat germ, dairy products, and egg yolk. To avoid deficiency, supplementation may be needed to improve interferon-gamma, interleukin 2, tumor necrosis factor and natural killer (NK) cell activity for improved immune function. Research from Dr. Bruce Ames, PhD, indicates that when cells fall short on any one of a handful of nutrients including zinc, severe genetic damages from mutations in the DNA and mitochondria occur [39]. Zinc is an important trace mineral needing careful monitoring following bariatric surgery [40].

Copper

Copper is essential for many enzymatic reactions in addition to its vital role in wound healing and immune function. Copper is an important factor in heme synthesis, melanin formation, and bone mineralization [7, pp. 159–161]. Absorption of copper occurs in the small intestine but gastric acid flow from the stomach is needed to enhance copper uptake [41].

Rats fed a copper-deficient diet develop lipid disorders with increased inflammatory issues [42]. Griffith et al. describe severe copper deficiency in two Roux-en-Y gastric bypass (RYGB) patients presenting with gait abnormalities and anemia. Intravenous and oral copper supplementation led to a resolution of anemia. The malabsorptive nature of bariatric surgery requires that the risk of copper deficiency be monitored throughout the patient's life.

Major food sources of copper include fish, meat, poultry, eggs, and nuts. Multivitamin and mineral supplementation may not be adequate for bariatric patients because of the copper to zinc ratio. Zinc interferes with copper absorption which has been shown to increase anemia, neutropenia, immune dysregulation, and lipid abnormalities in patients 2–10 years postsurgery [7, p. 161].

Survey

A national survey of dietary supplement recommendations pointed out the lack of research and clinical efficacy in England [44]. The time has come for more research on nutritional recommendations and rating of bariatric surgery success on nutritional well-being instead of pounds lost.

Nutrition Supplement Order Form

At the very least, a nutrition supplement order form should be provided to the patient pre- and postsurgery to impress on them the importance of adding nutrition to their dietary regime. A multivitamin and mineral capsule for use presurgery and opened up capsule after surgery + probiotic capsule + eicosapentaenoic acid–docosahexaenoic acid (EPA–DHA) gel cap should be recommended. Liquid forms are available for postsurgery incorporation into smoothies or soft food.

References

1. FDA. Warning letter. Available at: http://www.fda.gov/ICE-CI/Enforce mentActions/WarningLetters/2013/ucm349017.htm, March 19, 2013.
2. Flum DR, Salem I, Elrod JA, et al. Early mortality among Medicare beneficiaries undergoing bariatric surgical procedures. *JAMA* 2005;294: 1903–1908.

3. Still C, Sarwer DB, Blankenship J, eds. *The ASMBS Textbook of Bariatric Surgery*, vol 2. New York, NY: Springer-Verlag, 2014, p. 83.

4. Scheier L. Bariatric surgery: Life threatening risk or life-saving procedure? *J Am Diet Assn* 2004;104(9):1338–1340.

5. Tucker ME. Proper nutrition key following bariatric surgery. *Internal Med News* 37:22. Retrieved on Oct 27, 2010.

6. Lovett RA. Six more dietary ingredients picked for analytical evaluation. *Nutraceuticals World* 2016.

7. Gaby, AR. *Nutritional Medicine*. Concord, NH: Fritz Perlberg Publishing, 2011, pp. 89–96.

8. Pacholok SM, Stuart JJ. *Could It Be B12? An Epidemic of Misdiagnoses*. Fresno, CA: Quill Driver Books, 2011.

9. Doscherholmen A, McMahon J, Ripley D. Vitamin B12 assimilation from chicken meat. *Am J Clin Nutr* 1978;31:825–830.

10. Carmel B. Cobalamin (Vitamin B12). In Shils ME, Shike M, Ross AC, et al. eds. *Modern Nutrition in Health and Disease*, Tenth Edition. Baltimore, MD: Lippincott Williams & Wilkins, 2006, pp. 482–497.

11. Abdulla M, Anderson I, Asp NG, et al. Nutrient intake and health status of vegans. Chemical analyses of diets using duplicate portion sampling technique. *Am J Clin Nutr* 1981;34:2464–2477.

12. King CE, Leibach J, Toskes PP. Clinically significant vitamin B12 deficiency secondary to malabsorption of protein-bound vitamin B12. *Dig Dis Sci* 1979;24:397–402.

13. CDC. *National Report on Biochemical Indicators of Diet and Nutrition in the U.S. Population 1999-2002*, 2008. Available at: www.cdc.gov.

14. Lewerin C, Nilsson-Ehle H, Matousek M, et al. Reduction of plasma homocysteine and methylmalonate concentrations in apparently healthy elderly subjects after treatment with folic acid, vitamin B12 and vitamin B6: A randomized trial. *Eur J Clin Nutr* 2003;57:1426–1436.

15. Elia M. Oral or parenteral therapy for B12 deficiency. *Lancet* 1998;352:1721–1722.

16. Moore CE, Sherman V. Effectiveness of B vitamin supplementation following bariatric surgery: Rapid increases of serum B12. *Obes Surg* 2015;25:694–699.

17. Kassarjian Z, Russell RM. Hypochlorhydria: A factor in nutrition. *Annu Rev Nutr* 1989;9:271–285.

18. Menke A, Weimann HJ, Achtert G, et al. [Absolute bioavailability of folic acid after oral administration of a folic acid tablet formation in healthy volunteers]. *Arzneimittelforschung* 1994;44:1063–1067. [Translated from German.]

19. Babu S, Srikantia SG. Availability of folates from some foods. *Am J Clin Nutr* 1976;29:376–379.

20. Howard JS III. Folate deficiency in psychiatric practice. *Psychosomatics* 1975;16:112–115.

21. Elsborg L. Reversible malabsorption of folic acid in the elderly with nutritional folate deficiency. *Acta Haematol* 1976;55:140–147.

22. Leichter J, Landymore AF, Krumdieck CL. Folate conjugase activity in fresh vegetables and its effect on the determination of free folate content. *Am J Clin Nutr* 1979;32:92–95.

23. Whitney E, Rolfes SR. *Understanding Nutrition*. Belmont, CA: Wadsworth Publishing, 2008, pp. 334–337.

24. Holick MK. Vitamin D deficiency: What a pain it is. *Mayo Clin Proc* 2003;78:1457–1459.

25. Lee P, Greenfield JR, Seibel MJ, et al. Adequacy of Vitamin D replacement in severe deficiency is dependent on body mass index. *Am J Med* 2009;122:1056–1060.

26. Stokic E, Kupusinac A, Tomic-Naglic D, et al. Vitamin D and dysfunctional adipose tissue in obesity. *Angiology* 2015 Aug;66(7):613–618.

27. Ish-Shalom S, Segal E, Salganik T et al. Comparison of daily, weekly and monthly Vitamin D3 in ethanol dosing protocols for two months in elderly hip fracture patients. *J Clin Endocrinol Metab* 2008;93:3430–3435.

28. Hollik MK. Vitamin D deficiency. *New England J Med* 2007;357(3): 266–281.

29. USDA UV-B Monitoring and Research Program at Colorado State University. Available at: uvb.nrel.colostate.edu/UVB.

30. Chan L, Neilson CH, Kirk EA, et al. Optimization of Vitamin D status after Roux-en-Y gastric bypass surgery in obese patients living in northern climate. *Obes Surg* 2015;25:2321–2327.

31. Shearer MJ. Vitamin K. *Lancet* 1995; 245:229–234.

32. Rucker RB. Improved functional endpoints for use in Vitamin K assessment: important implications for bone disease. *Am J Clin Nutr* 1997;65:883–884.

33. Krasinski SD, Russell RM, Furie BC, et al. The prevalence of Vitamin K deficiency in chronic gastrointestinal disorders. *Am J Clin Nutr* 1985;41:639–643.

34. Kadrabova J, Madaric A, Kovacikova Z, et al. Selenium status, plasma zinc, copper and magnesium in vegetarians. *Biol Trac Elem Res* 1995;50:13–24.

35. Alasfar F, Ben-Nakhi M, Khoursheed M, et al. Selenium is significantly depleted among morbidly obese female patients seeking bariatric surgery. *Obes Surg* 2011;21:1710–1713.

36. Bales CW, Steinman LC, Freeland-Graves JH, et al. The effect of age on plasma zinc uptake and taste acuity. *Am J Clin Nutr* 1986;44:664–669.

37. Prasad AS. Clinical and biochemical manifestations of zinc deficiency in human subjects. *Am Coll Nutr* 1985;4:65–72.

38. Pfeiffer CC, Jenny EH. Fingernail white spots: Possible zinc deficiency. *JAMA* 1974;228:157.

39. Jaret P. The Ames Prescription. *Alternative Medicine* June 2005.

40. Billeter AT, Probst P, Fischer L, et al. Risk of malnutrition, trace metal, and vitamin deficiency post Roux-en-Y gastric bypass- a prospective study of 20 patients with BMI <35 kg/m². *Obes Surg* 2015;25:2125–2134.

41. Tompsett SL. Factors influencing the absorption of iron and copper from the alimentary tract. *Biochem J* 1940;34:961–69.

42. Kramer TR, Johnson WT, Briske-Anerson MJ, et al. Copper deficiency and rat spleen lymphocyte biology. *Fed Proc* 1985;44:1150.

43. Griffith DP, Liff D, Ziegler TR et al. Acquired copper deficiency: a potentially serious and preventable complication following gastric bypass surgery. *Obesity* 2009 April;17(4):827–831.

44. Dunstan MJD, Molena EJ, et al. Variations in oral vitamin and mineral supplementation following bariatric gastric bypass surgery: A national survey. *Obes Surg* 2015;25:648–55.

7

Post-op Discharge Diets

Diet modifications following surgery focus on texture, consistency, and frequency of eating to insure nutritional adequacy and tolerance. Nutrition monitoring following surgery is an important factor in weight loss success and quality of life.

Diet Stages Roux-En-Y Gastric Bypass and Sleeve Gastrectomy

Stage 1: Days 1 and 2	Clear Liquids: sips of water hourly (1 oz./hr day 1, 2 oz./hr day 2). Sugar-free popsicles and room temperature chicken broth may also be consumed NO: carbonated beverages, high-sugar drinks, coffee, tea, energy drinks
Stage 2: Days 3–10	Full Liquids: Continue clear liquids (3–4 oz./hr). Advance to protein smoothies using yogurt or kefir. Sugar-free gelatin for hydration. Cream of chicken soup (no chunks). Eat 3–5 times/day Consume 48–60 oz. fluid/day NO: carbonated beverages but "flat" diet beverages may be consumed for hydration
Stage 3: Days 11–21	Puree with high-protein smoothies: Pureed chicken in soup, mashed tuna with mayo, cottage cheese with pureed peaches, protein smoothies, creamed soups, sugar-free popsicles Eat 3–5 times/day. NO: fluids with meals Consume 48–60 oz. fluid/day
Stage 4: Days 22–30	Soft Cooked Foods: Scrambled egg, pureed/chopped turkey or chicken or pork, cooked

	vegetables, ripe avocado, cooked or frozen pureed fruit, coffee/tea
	Continue protein smoothies
	Eat 5–6 times/day. NO: fluids with meals.
Stage 5*: 1–2 months	Advance diet as tolerated. Cooked soft meats, steamed vegetables, soft peeled fresh fruit (banana)
	Eat 5–6 times/day. NO: fluids with meals
	No: bread, pasta, rice, beans/legumes, high-fructose corn sweeteners, carbonated beverages, alcoholic beverages
Stage 6	Diet as tolerated with adequate protein at each meal time
	Controlled portions. Raw salads are not encouraged—they may be tolerated but provide poor-quality protein and displace other quality proteins.

A study by Arvidsson et al. indicated that patients did not need to refrain from drinking during meals the first year after Roux-en-Y gastric bypass (RYGB) [1].

Diet Stages Laparoscopic Adjustable Gastric Banding

Stages 1 and 2 are same as RYGB and sleeve gastrectomy (SG).

Stage 3: Days 11–14	Puree with high-protein smoothies. Pureed chicken in soup, mashed tuna with mayo, cottage cheese with pureed peaches, protein smoothies, creamed soups, sugar-free popsicles
	Eat 3–5 times/day. NO: fluids with meals
	Consume 48–60 oz. fluid/day
Stage 4: Days 15–30	Soft Cooked Foods: Scrambled egg, pureed/chopped turkey or chicken or pork, cooked vegetables, ripe avocado, cooked or frozen

---

* Nutritional assessment labs to appraise pre-albumin, albumin, anemia, Vitamin D.

	pureed fruit, coffee/tea. Continue protein smoothies
	Eat 3–5 times/day. NO: fluids with meals.
Stage 5: 1–2 months	Diet as tolerated: well cooked, soft meats, cooked vegetables, soft fresh, or frozen fruits (no peels or seeds)
	Eat 3–5 times/day. High-protein food at each meal. No fluids with meals
Stage 6: Laparoscopic adjustable gastric banding (LAGB) fill	Full liquid diet 1–2 days postfill before advancing as tolerated

Nutrition and Bariatric Surgery [2] and the *ASMBS Textbook of Bariatric Surgery* [3] provide similar surgery staging protocols for RYGB, SG, and LAGB.

Carbonated Beverages

Carbonated beverages are discouraged because they may cause gas to be trapped in the anastomoses where the stomach pouch meets the small intestine. This gas not only creates discomfort but could also stretch the connection and, therefore, cause decreased feeling of fullness which will affect weight loss after the RYGB surgery.

Dumping Syndrome

Dumping syndrome is mainly a concern for RYGB patients who do not have a pyloric sphincter to regulate high-sugar foods that create a hypertonic response in the jejunum. As early as 10–13 minutes after eating the high-sugar food, the patient can get abdominal cramps and diarrhea or a feeling of dizziness and lightheadedness [4,5].

The dumping syndrome response to hyperosmolar meals is a problem in bariatric surgery patients because the pyloric sphincter would normally control the rate of flow from the stomach into the duodenum. After RYGB, the hypertonic gastric contents can rush into the small intestine after eating. Early symptoms can occur within minutes due to large fluid shift from blood plasma to the intestines and the increase in peristaltic activity of the gut. Several hours later symptoms of hypoglycemia may occur because of the high-blood-glucose spike and excessive insulin response [6].

Limiting the quantity of food and carbohydrate levels can minimize or prevent dumping syndrome. Fluids are restricted during meals and sugars—including lactose—are restricted or limited to control symptoms. Eating slowly and chewing thoroughly while sitting upright can also help reduce symptoms [7].

GERD or Gastroesophageal Reflux Disease

GERD or commonly called reflux esophagitis is an inflammation caused from gastric juice flowing into the esophagus. The reflux of acidic gastric juice into the lower end of the esophagus erodes the mucosal lining of the esophagus. Changes in the height of the basal cell layer and the papillae can stimulate nerves that are sensitive to acid like orange juice, or aspirin passing through the esophagus, which causes a heartburn sensation [8,9].

The main function of the esophagus is to carry food from the mouth to the cardia of the stomach. The cardia normally prevents leakage of the gastric juices back into the esophagus from the stomach and its major role is to allow belching of gases consumed from carbonated beverages or fermented products like beer [10].

Treatment for GERD is usually with histamine blockers or omeprazole. Individuals prone to GERD should be advised to avoid foods that are known to increase symptoms of reflux like chocolate, peppermint, onions, coffee, alcohol, and fatty foods [11].

Hypoglycemia

Post-RYGB surgery, patients may experience hypoglycemia as a result of food dumping quickly into the small intestine causing hyperglycemia and the insulin response. In severe cases, this could cause the patient to pass out. This syndrome does not occur in patients who have their pylorus intact—adjustable gastric banding or vertical SG— according to John P. Bantle, MD, endocrinologist and professor of medicine at the University of Minnesota, Minneapolis [12].

Carbohydrate restriction or avoidance is the best treatment for RYGB patients who report this syndrome. Patients who need a quick solution to hypoglycemia should have one or two glucose pills ready to take at the first sign of any hypoglycemia.

Rariy et al. reported on postgastric bypass hypoglycemia in the February 2016 issue of *Current Diabetes Report*. He indicated that despite the benefits of bariatric surgery, hypoglycemic complications are something that physicians and health-care personnel need to be aware of as more patients use bariatric surgery to control their weight [13].

Avoid Fluids with Meals

After surgery it is important not to drink fluids with meals and up to 30 minutes after meals. Drinking fluids during a meal or soon after flushes food through too fast and can cause regurgitation. High-carbohydrate foods like juices, ice cream, fast food milkshakes, and sodas go down quickly but can cause bloating and nausea, in addition to not being good for weight loss.

Encourage Eating Slowly and Chewing Thoroughly

Once the liquid diet stage is passed, patients need to relearn how to eat slowly and mindfully. They need to start by taking a pencil eraser size bite of scrambled egg or cottage cheese and chewing it thoroughly. Keeping the food in the mouth until it is a liquid consistency is important for digestion and bioavailability of nutrients from the food. Mindful eating means they stop eating when they feel full.

Mindful Eating

Long-term success for a bariatric surgery patient depends on lifestyle changes that include mindful and sustainable new eating habits, along with physical activity and nutrition repletion. People hate counting calories and being scolded when they splurge on the wrong foods. Each patient needs to make peace with food and get support to reinvigorate their healthy food choices in order to prevent regaining weight.

Medical professionals seldom learn about the satiety and physiological mechanisms that influence food intake. Appetite is a multiphase process occurring numerous times a day for an individual and it influences the desire to eat. Hunger is the primary component of appetite. Satiety is the feeling achieved when the need for energy has been fulfilled.

Hormonal regulation controls much of the digestive process with ghrelin signaling the brain to eat based on smell, sight of food, or to maintain energy. Cholecystokinin (CCK) also signals satiation by activating receptors to reduce gastric emptying by the pyloric sphincter. Proteins and complex carbohydrates effectively stimulate CCK while a meal rich in glucose or lactose does not [14].

Glucose-dependent insulinotropic polypeptide (GIP) is released within 5 minutes after food ingestion and peaks 30–60 minutes later, depending on the meal size and composition. Mans et al. found that SG accelerated gastric emptying, enhanced CCK and GIP levels, plus reduced ghrelin release which helped patients lose weight and improve their glucose metabolism [15]. GIP regulates pancreatic secretions like insulin and lipase for carbohydrate and lipid metabolism.

Gastric motility is stimulated by food moving through the digestive tract and signaling release of digestive enzymes like peptide tyrosine–tyrosine (PYY) and glucagon-like peptide (GLP-1). Yan et al. reported that meal size had a significant impact on PYY and GLP-1 secretion after RYGB [16]. Meal sizes, as small as 75–300 kcal, were significantly effective in increasing levels of these peptides and affecting weight loss. Both PYY and GLP-1 are released by intestinal enteroendocrine cells and have a role in reducing gastric motility and probably appetite.

Crosstalk between GIP and GLP-1 is speculated since carbohydrates influence pancreatic insulin hormone release, and PYY assists in reducing motility so brakes can be applied to allow satiety signal transmission to the brain [14].

There were no major differences in food preferences or intake between RYGB and SG groups studied by El Labban [17]. However, a trend in eating sweets by SG subjects was identified. Mindful eating means cutting added sugars which add no micronutrients to the diet. Eating for health instead of consuming sweets and fatty foods requires discipline. As Ferris Jabr wrote in *Scientific American*, "extremely sweet or fatty foods captivate the brain's reward circuit in much the same way that cocaine and gambling do" [18].

Gluten

Gluten is a protein found in wheat, barley, and rye grains that can create intolerance and gut problems for individuals sensitive to the protein. The food industry has capitalized on gluten-free options for meals and many restaurants even offer a gluten-free menu.

Celiac disease affects about 1% of the population and is an auto-immune disease. Many weight loss patients have used the "gluten-free" way in their attempt to lose weight and many of them report feeling better with less gastrointestinal (GI) bloating and gas.

Going gluten-free is not harmful but bariatric patients need to be reminded that many of these products contain high levels of simple carbohydrates making them off limits in a ketogenic diet.

Lactose Intolerance

Milk and milk products—including caseinate supplements—can cause gas, abdominal bloating, or diarrhea. As the undigested lactose milk sugar moves through the GI tract, these symptoms can lead to vomiting and severe pain. Most mammals cease producing lactase, the enzyme needed to digest lactose, soon after weaning but persistence of drinking milk or eating ice cream into adulthood can produce a tolerance until physiological responses change. Avoidance of dairy products or selection of fermented ones like cheese, yogurt, or kefir can reduce symptoms [19].

Lactulose is not lactose but many people do not know there is a difference. Lactose is a sugar that can raise blood glucose. Lactulose is a synthetic sugar that is broken down in the colon and removed from the body in the feces. Because lactulose pulls water out of the body and into the colon, GI issues like diarrhea and bloating may be experienced from eating foods containing it.

Food Sensitivities

Although some physicians recognize classical food allergies commonly referred to as IgE mediated, adverse food reactions or food sensitivities of IgG response can cause numerous symptoms that bariatric surgery patients may present with. The practitioner may have problems identifying a particular food(s) that cause(s) adverse reactions but convenient diagnostic blood tests are available to aid in the diagnosis, which leads to eliminating or limiting the trigger foods from the diet.

Typical food allergens include milk, peanuts, shellfish, eggs, soy, wheat, tree nuts, and fish [20]. IgE allergic reactions are often quick to develop and can be life threatening such as acute asthma or anaphylaxis [21]. Food sensitivity or intolerance or "hidden" food allergy is often associated with GI symptoms that may not disappear as a result of bariatric surgery. The fast acting immunoglobulin E antibodies against an offending food involves an intensive fast attack whereas, food sensitivity symptoms can take hours or days to develop and can come and go in cycles or seasons [22].

A food elimination diet based on IgG antibody testing results can be an effective and targeted approach to reduce food intolerance symptoms of migraines, Crohn's disease, irritable bowel syndrome (IBS), arthritis, and asthma. Diagnostic testing is available at several laboratories using a biochemical method known as the enzyme-linked immunosorbent assay (ELISA).

Alcohol Consumption

Ethanol alters the metabolism of protein, fat, and carbohydrates. It inhibits plasma protein and complement synthesis so its allowance in the diet of a bariatric surgery patient increases the risk of malnutrition. As Di Salvo reports, alcohol affects the brain and the body through its effect on neurotransmitters [23]. He outlines the alcohol reward effect with a clear explanation as to why alcohol abuse among postoperative bariatric patients is so widely reported [24–27].

Steffen et al. provide new information on the rapid rate of absorption of alcohol after RYGB. They report that within minutes after consumption, a RYGB patient achieves a very high-blood alcohol concentration that could affect legal driving limits [28].

Caffeine Concerns

Caffeine (1,3,7-trimethylxanthine) has been consumed in coffee, tea, and chocolate for hundreds of years and soft drinks for more than 120 years [29]. Caffeine content of foods and beverages varies with the type of product and the method of preparation with the major sources of caffeine in the American diet being coffee, soft drinks, and tea [30]. Caffeine is rapidly absorbed from the GI tract and metabolized in the liver.

Ground roasted coffee contains 85 mg caffeine per 5 oz. and is the primary source of caffeine in the diet. Instant coffee has 60 mg caffeine per 5 oz. and decaffeinated coffee equals 3 mg caffeine in a 5 oz. cup. Colas are the second most consumed source of caffeine with 18 mg per 6 oz. serving. Black tea contains 30 mg per 5 oz. steeped cup or 20 mg per 5 oz. serving of instant tea. Chocolate/cocoa has 4 mg per 5 oz. serving.

Caffeine has been reported in numerous studies to have ergogenic affects to increase athletic performance, endurance, and mental clarity but for bariatric patients, detrimental effects, such as gastric upset, withdrawal symptoms, sleep disturbance, and interaction with mineral supplements can outweigh the benefits.

Attention on safety of caffeine has been focused on energy drinks and beverages that contain caffeine and other stimulants. The Food and Drug Administration (FDA) and Centers for Disease Control and Prevention (CDC) have warned about the dangers of mixing alcohol and energy drinks because the high amounts of caffeine in the energy drinks can mask the intoxicating effects of alcohol while having no effect on alcohol metabolism, which could increase the risk of alcohol-related injuries [30].

Caffeine is not recommended during early stages of post-op bariatric surgery because of its effect on the central nervous system. The stimulating effects of caffeine could affect blood pressure, disrupt sleep, and exacerbate psychiatric conditions.

Coffee has been called "chemistry in a cup" because it contains almost 2,000 compounds [31]. *The Journal of Agricultural and Food Chemistry* reports that dark roast coffee produces a chemical that helps prevent the production of excess stomach acid [32] and another study [33] in 2011 found that coffee led to significant body weight reduction in preobese volunteers. That may help bariatric surgery patients decide whether to include coffee in their diet.

For many, making coffee is a morning routine. It is much easier to make bad coffee than good coffee with health benefits. For the most nutritive benefits, grind the coffee beans just before brewing to get the best flavor and healthy polyphenols. Ground coffee loses flavor and nutrient benefits upon exposure to air.

Tea use has been associated with improved cognition according to a study in the *American Journal of Clinical Nutrition* [34] with green tea offering high levels of catechin (antioxidants). The polyphenol L-theanine in tea has neuroprotective effects for calming and stress reduction.

The methylxanthine in cocoa or theobromine as some biochemists like to call it, can have detrimental effects for those with GERD and migraines [35].

Nutritional Deficiency

Bariatric surgery is able to provide a better quality of life for many obese individuals, however, it comes with complications of malnutrition. Peterson et al. found malnutrition in bariatric surgery candidates **prior** to surgery that were correlated with adverse surgical outcomes [36]. Up to 4.7% of the patients in a study by Faintuch et al. were reported to have protein-calorie malnutrition [37]. Numerous nutritional deficiency reports abound in the medical literature [38–44].

Nutrient deficiencies were not only found in RYGB. The SG and adjustable gastric banding research also indicated severe nutrient depletion for Vitamin B_{12}, folate, and Vitamin D [45–47].

Food or Pills

There are many factors that influence nutrient uptake and utilization. Mechanisms that regulate the absorption or excretion of nutrients in a bariatric patient depend on a host of factors—age, sex, physiological state—in addition to dietary sources and its nutrient content. Plant foods contain phytates, oxalates, and polyphenols, which reduce absorption of nutrients from them. There is much to learn about the analytical versus biological dietetics aspect of food. Many questions remain about bioavailability of food components and their effect on the microbiome. Bariatric surgery creates even more consequences. Are the innate nutrients in food better than those found in dietary supplements? As Roger Clemens, Doctor of Public Health, Chief Scientific Officer, Horn Company, LeMirada, CA states, "At this juncture of our understanding of nutrient bioavailability, it just depends" [48].

References

1. Arvidsson A, Evertsson I, Ekelund M, et al. Water with food intake does not influence caloric intake after gastric bypass (GBP): A cross-over trial. *Obes Surg* 2015;25:249–253.
2. Cummings S. Nutrition management, pre-and post surgery. Kushner RF, Still CD, eds. *Nutrition and Bariatric Surgery*. Boca Raton, FL: CRC Press, 2015, pp. 33–53.
3. Lewis FL. Perioperative nutritional assessment of the bariatric surgery patient. In: Still CD, Sarwer DB, eds. *The ASMBS Textbook of Bariatric Surgery*, vol 2. New York, NY: Springer, 2014, pp. 77–87.
4. Del Valle. Peptic ulcer disease and related disorders. In: Longo DL, Fauci AS, Kasper DL, et al., eds. *Harrison's Principles of Internal Medicine*, Eighteenth Edition. New York, NY: McGraw-Hill, 2014.
5. NIH—National Institute of Diabetes and Digestive and Kidney Diseases. Dumping Syndrome. Available at www.niddk.nih.gov.
6. Rolfes SR, Pinna K, Whitney E. *Understanding Normal and Clinical Nutrition*. Belmont, CA: Wadsworth Publishing, Thomson Learning, 2006, pp. 727–730.
7. Nguyen NQ, Debrecceni TL, Burgstad CM, et al. Effects of posture and meal volume on gastric emptying, intestinal transit, oral glucose tolerance, blood pressure, and gastrointestinal symptoms after Roux-en-Y Gastric Bypass. *Obes Surg* 2015;25:1392–1400.
8. Spiro HM. *Clinical Gastroenterolgy*. New York, NY: McGraw-Hill, 2002.
9. Sitaraman S, Friedman LS, eds. Essentials of Gastroenterology. Oxford, UK: John Wiley & Sons, 2012.
10. Goldstein JL, Schlesinger PK, Mozwecz HL, et al. Esophageal mucosal resistance. A factor in esophagitis. *Gastroenterol Clin N Amer* 1990;19:565.
11. Kitchin LI, Castell DO. Rationale and efficacy of conservative therapy for gastroesophageal reflux disease. *Arch Intern Med* 1991;151:448.
12. ADA. Advanced Postgraduate Course. San Francisco, CA: ADA, 2016.
13. Rariy CM, Rometo D Korytkowski M. Post-gastric bypass hypoglycemia. *Curr Diab Rep* 2016 Feb;16(2):12.
14. Paeschke TM, Aimutis WR. Formulating for satiety with hydrocolloids. *Food Technology* 2011 Mar;24–32.
15. Mans E, Serra-Prat M, Palomera E, et al. Sleeve gastrectomy effects on hunger, satiation, and gastrointestinal hormone and motility responses after a liquid meal test. *Am J Clin Nutr* 2015;102:540–547.
16. Yan W, Polidori D, Yieh L, et al. Effects of meal size on the release of GLP-1 and PYY after Roux-en-Y gastric bypass surgery in obese subjects with or without type 2 diabetes. *Obes Surg* 2014;24:1969–1974.
17. El Labban S, Safadi B, Olabi A. The effect of Roux-en-Y gastric bypass and sleeve gastrectomy surgery on dietary intake, food preferences, and gastrointestinal symptoms in post surgical morbidly obese Lebanese subjects: A cross-sectional pilot study. *Obes Surg* 2015;25:2393–2399.

18. Jabr F. That craving for dessert. *Scientific American* 2016 Jan;314:23–24.
19. Savaiano DA, Levitt MD. Milk intolerance and microbe-containing dairy foods. *J Dairy Sci* 1987;70(2):397–406.
20. Gaby AR. The role of hidden food allergy/intolerance in chronic disease. *Altern Med Rev* 1998 Apr;3(2):90–100.
21. Wuthrich B. [Food allergy, food intolerance or functional disorder?] [Article in German] *Praxis (Bern 1994)* 2009 Apr 1;98(7):375–387.
22. Patriarca G, Schiavino D, Pecora V, et al. Food allergy and food intolerance: diagnosis and treatment. *Intern Emerg Med* 2009 Feb;4(1):11–24.
23. DiSalvo D. What does alcohol do to your brain? *Forbes.* Oct 2012.
24. Spadola CE, Wagner EF, Dillon FR, et al. Alcohol and drug use among post operative bariatric patients: A systematic review of the emerging research and its implications. *Alcohol Clin Exp Res* 2015 Sep;39(9):1582–1601.
25. Svensson PA, Anveden A, Romeo S, et al. Alcohol consumption and alcohol problems after bariatric surgery in the Swedish obese subjects study. *Obesity* 2013; 21(12):244–251.
26. Burgos MG, Cabral PC, Maio R, et al. Prevalence of alcohol abuse before and after bariatric surgery associated with nutrition and lifestyle factors: A study involving a Portuguese population. *Obes Surg* 2015;25(9):1716–1722.
27. Steffen KJ, Engel SG, Wonderlich JA, et al. Alcohol and other additive disorders following bariatric surgery: Prevalence, risk factors and possible etiologies. *Eur Eat Disord Rev* 2015;23(6):442–450.
28. Steffen KJ, Engel SG, et al. Blood alcohol concentrations rise rapidly and dramatically after Roux-en-Y gastric bypass. *Surg Obes Relat Dis* 2013;9(3): 470–473.
29. Heckman MA, Weil J, Gonzalez de Mejia E, et al. Caffeine (1, 3, 7-trimethylxanthine) in foods: A comprehensive review on consumption, functionality, safety, and regulatory matters. *J Food Sci* 2010Apr;75 (3):R77–87.
30. Memelstein NH. Caffeinated concerns. *Food Technology* May 2015; 69–71.
31. Clemens R, Hayes AW, Kruger C. Understanding the difference between hazard and risk. *Food Technol* 2016 Jan;1(16):18-19.
32. Rubach M, Lang R, Skupin C, et al. Activity-guided fractionation to characterize a coffee beverage that effectively down-regulates mechanisms of gastric acid secretion as compared to regular coffee. *J. Agric. Food Chem* 2010;58(7):4153-4161.
33. Kotyczka C, Boettler U, Lang R, et al. Dark roast coffee is more effective than light roast coffee in reducing body weight and in restoring red blood cell Vitamin E and glutathione concentrations in healthy volunteers. *Mol Nutr Food Res* 2011 Oct; 55(10):1582-1586.
34. Ng TP, Feng L, Niti M et al. Tea consumption and cognitive impairment and decline in older Chinese adults. *Am J Clin Nutr* 2008; 88:224-231.
35. Shively CA, Tarka Sm. Methylxanthine composition and consumption patterns of cocoa and chocolate products. *Prog Clin Biol Res* 1984;158:149-178.

36. Peterson LA, Cheskin LJ, Furtado M, et al. Malnutrition in bariatric surgery candidates: Multiple micronutrient deficiencies prior to surgery. *Obes Surg* 2016 Apr; 26(4):833–838.

37. Faintuch J, Matsuda M, Cruz ME, et al. Severe protein-calorie malnutrition after bariatric procedures. *Obes Surg* 2004;14:175–181.

38. Muschitz C, Kocijan R, Haschka J, et al. The impact of vitamin D, calcium, protein supplementation, and physical exercise on bone metabolism after bariatric surgery: The BABS study. *J Bone Miner Res* 2016 Mar;31:672–682.

39. Billeter ATY, Probst P, Fischer L, et al. Risk of malnutrition, trace metal and vitamin deficiency post Roux-en-Y gastric bypass—A prospective study of 20 patients with BMI < 35 kg/m². *Obes Surg* 2015;25:2125–2134.

40. Gong K, Gagner M, Pomp A, et al. Micronutrient deficiencies after laparoscopic gastric bypass: Recommendations. *Obes Surg* 2008;18:1062–1066.

41. Van der Beek ES, Monpellier VM, Eland I, et al. Nutritional deficiencies in gastric bypass patients; incidence, time of occurrence and implications for post-operative surveillance. *Obes Surg* 2015;25:818–823.

42. Schweitzer DH, Posthuma EF. Prevention of vitamin and mineral deficiencies after bariatric surgery: evidence and algorithms. *Obes Surg* 2008;18:1485–1488.

43. Davies DJ, Baxter JN. Nutritional deficiencies after bariatric surgery. *Obes Surg* 2007;17:1150–1158.

44. Xanthakos SA. Nutritional deficiencies in obesity after bariatric surgery. *Pediatr Clin North Am* 2009;56:1105–1121.

45. Van Rutte PWJ, Aarts EO, Smulders JF, et al. Nutrient deficiencies before and after sleeve gastrectomy. *Obes Surg* 2014;24:1639–1646.

46. Coupaye M, Riviere P, Breuil MC, et al. Comparison of nutritional status during the first year after sleeve gastrectomy and Roux-en-Y gastric bypass. *Obes Surg* 2014;24: 276–283.

47. Coupaye M, Puchaux K, et al. Nutritional consequences of adjustable gastric banding and gastric bypass: A 1 year prospective study. *Obes Surg* 2009;19:56–65.

48. Clemons R. Which is best: food or dietary supplements? *Food Technology.* Jan 2015, p. 17.

8

METABOLIC CONCERNS AND BARIATRIC SURGERY

Bariatric surgery may pose a significant opportunity and challenge for individuals who have underlying metabolic conditions that contributed to their obesity—hyperglycemia, hyperinsulinemia, hypertriglyceridemia, hypercholesterolemia, insulin resistance, hypothyroidism, polycystic ovary syndrome (PCOS), and genetic factors like methylene tetrahydrofolate reductase (MTHFR). Obesity results from the following five basic etiologies, according to Plaisted and Istfan [1]:

- Hyperphagia—abnormally increased appetite for consumption of food associated with injury to hypothalamus
- Reduced physical activity
- Endocrine disorders—adrenal, thyroid
- Sympathetic nervous system dysfunction—hypertension
- Dysinsulinemia—enhanced adipose deposition

Obesity predisposes an individual to cardiovascular risk factors such as dyslipidemia, type 2 diabetes (T2DM), nonalcoholic fatty liver disease (NAFLD), and hypertension [2]. Roux-en-Y gastric bypass (RYGB)-induced sustained weight loss can result in metabolic improvement compared with pharmacological interventions.

Dyslipidemia

Blood lipids are strongly associated with body size and adiposity. Hypertriglyceridemia may result from the overproduction of very low-density lipoprotein (VLDL) and many patients with elevated triglycerides also have insulin resistance that causes the overproduction of VLDL [3]. Hypercholesterolemia is also common in obesity, which manifests as elevated low-density lipoprotein (LDL). Calorie excess raises hepatic synthesis of lipoproteins and results in glucose intolerance [4].

Bariatric surgery resulted in significant weight loss that has a marked effect on serum lipid levels as reported by Feingold et al. [5]. The low-carbohydrate diet pre- and postsurgery decreases triglyceride levels to a greater extent than high-carbohydrate diets, and produces marked weight loss differences. The human lipoprotein kinetic study of 2014 showed the effects of bariatric surgery on triglyceride-rich lipoproteins in decreasing cardiovascular mortality after surgery [6].

Batsis et al. reported on bariatric surgery improvement of cardiovascular risk factors in a geriatric population with significant reductions in weight, diabetes, hypertension, dyslipidemia, and sleep apnea [7]. Weight loss at 6 months postbariatric surgery produced an effective reduction in cardiovascular disease, diabetes, and related mortality as observed in a short-term study by Domienik-Karlowicz et al. [8] and management survey of endocrine diseases by Corcellas et al. [9].

Laparoscopic sleeve gastrectomy (LSG) weight loss improved levels of C-reactive proteins—markers of inflammation—dyslipidemia, and cancer antigen-125 (CA-125), linked to obesity and tumors [10].

Hyperglycemia

Patients with prediabetes and obesity need nutrition therapy but seldom receive it because it is an out-of-pocket expense. Prediabetes is a term used to convey that a person is at risk for diabetes with fasting blood glucose (FBG) of 100–125 mg/dL or 2-hour postprandial glucose level of 140–190 mg/dL [11]. Long-term use of antidepressant therapy and certain statin drugs can increase the risk of T2DM in the prediabetic population [11, p. 7].

Currently, metformin is the most widely prescribed antihyperglycemic agent and it is the first-line therapy for T2DM. Metformin lowers glucose by reducing the rate of hepatic glucose production, which can be significantly increased in T2DM due to poor food choices and inactivity. Since metformin does not cause hypoglycemia, it can safely be used in prediabetes, gestational diabetes, and PCOS [12].

The evaluation of gastric banding, gastric bypass, and sleeve gastrectomy in obtaining glycemic control is reviewed in numerous studies with the general outcome favoring gastric bypass and sleeve gastrectomy [13–20].

Cummings et al. conducted a trial known as Calorie Reduction or Surgery: Seeking Remission of Obesity and Diabetes (CROSSROADS) involving patients (body mass index [BMI]: 30–40) with T2DM. The benefits of bariatric surgery (gastric bypass) were significantly greater than medical and lifestyle interventions [21]. After 1 year, 60% of the gastric bypass patients were still in diabetes remission, whereas only 6% on the medical/lifestyle program were in remission. Weight loss was greater in the gastric bypass group than in the nonsurgical approach group at 1 year.

Although the mainstay of treatment for T2DM has been pharmacologic and lifestyle modification, glycemic control through bariatric surgery has been associated with remission of the disease [22–25].

But the majority of the studies supporting bariatric surgery and diabetes remission have only short-term follow-up. A long-term study showing remission rates greater than 5 years was reported by Brethauer et al. in 2013 with partial or complete remission achieved in a percentage of T2DM individuals [26]. Those diagnosed <5 years with T2DM had a 76% remission rate compared with those diagnosed >5 years, with a 21% remission rate.

According to Panunji et al. in *Diabetes Care*, the major determining factor for diabetes remission and glycemic control is weight loss [27]. Remission rates were reported from 37%–95% based on surgical weight loss versus medical therapy and lifestyle changes. Since the International Diabetes Federation guidelines indicate bariatric surgery for patients with a BMI >40, those with a BMI of 35–40 are usually limited to medical therapy and lifestyle changes with little hope of remission.

Weight loss was cited by numerous studies as the primary factor for hyperglycemia management [28–30] and every effort needs to be made to assist T2DM patients with an opportunity for an effective weigh loss regime.

Dietary management for hyperglycemia focuses on avoiding excess sugar intake, reducing processed foods, and adding dietary supplements like chromium, vanadium, berberine, and cinnamon to help improve glucose control and insulin sensitivity. Addressing the deeper cause of glucose elevation, like gut inflammation, also needs to be considered.

Skipping breakfast has been shown to increase HgbA1c (A1c) and cause all day postprandial hyperglycemia in patients with T2DM. The extended fasting period created by skipping breakfast leads to reduced insulin and glucagon-like peptide-1 (GLP-1) levels, which decreases the activation of beta cells. This disruption of the circadian clock leads to increased postprandial glucose after lunch and dinner in T2DM patients [31].

T2DM is a complex and multifaceted disease requiring lifestyle interventions to achieve glycemic control but a recent study in *JAMA* reported improvement is better postbariatric surgery than with just lifestyle changes so health-care professionals need to stress bariatric surgery as a tool along with lifestyle changes [32]. Another study compared RYGB surgery with laparoscopic gastric sleeve surgery and a control group receiving intensive lifestyle weight loss intervention. Forty percent of the RYGB patients and 29% of the gastric sleeve participants achieved partial or complete remission of T2DM. Partial remission was defined as FBG ≤125 mg/dL and A1c <6.5% without medication and complete remission defined as FBG ≤100 mg/dL and A1c <5.7%, without medication. None of the lifestyle only participants had remission [33].

The efficacy of bariatric surgery in the treatment of T2DM is demonstrated by marked improvements in insulin sensitivity within the first few days after RYGB even before weight loss has occurred. However, long-term postoperative effectiveness was inconclusive due to limited follow-up research [34].

Xiong et al. monitored fasting GLP-1 and 2-hour GLP-1 values in a T2DM population. RYGB patients showed significant increase in GLP-1 and decreased fasting glucose-dependent insulinotropic polypeptide (GIP), which lead to improved glycemic control [35].

An LSG study reported in *JAMA Surgery* [36] indicates weight loss of 77%, 70%, 56% during the 1, 3, and 5 years of study respectively, with maintenance of complete remission of diabetes in 51%, 38%, and 20%, respectively, during that period. Hypertension and dyslipidemia were also improved but a significant weight gain occurred with long-term LSG patients.

Type 1 diabetes mellitus is increasing globally and leading to increased morbidity and mortality from obesity. Bariatric surgery achieved a significant improvement in insulin requirements but had only a modest effect on glycemic control in studies by Ashrafian and Mahawar [37,38].

Nutritional management for glycemic control focuses on a high-protein diet resulting in reduced liver enzymes aspartate aminotransferase (AST), alanine aminotransferase (ALT) and gamma-glutamyltransferase (GGT) along with a lower A1c [39]. Many studies have focused on the effects of the Mediterranean diet [40] but a recent study has indicated that a Nordic diet also can reduce the risk of T2DM. The Nordic food index is composed of six foods: fish, cabbage, rye bread, oatmeal, apples, pears, and root vegetables [41].

NAFLD and Nonalcoholic Steatohepatitis

As previously mentioned, a high-protein diet provided a reduction in liver enzymes. Bariatric surgery has also been shown to have an improvement in NAFLD by reduction of inflammatory markers. Long-term studies on which type of surgery and if it is capable of curing the disease are lacking [42]. Clark et al. in 2005, reported improvement in NAFLD after RYGB surgery induced weight loss [43].

The prevalence of NAFLD and nonalcoholic steatohepatitis (NASH) in morbidly obese patients undergoing bariatric surgery appears to be associated with dyslipidemia according to Feijo et al. [44]. Another study, considered the prevalence of NAFLD among severely obese adolescents undergoing bariatric surgery who presented with ALT levels and cardiometabolic risk factors associated with abnormal immune function and lipid metabolism issues [45].

Both NAFLD and NASH are increasingly common causes of chronic liver disease worldwide. The effective treatment for NAFLD is weight reduction with sustained weight loss [46]. Obesity is the significant risk factor in the development of hepatic steatosis and NASH with development of hepatic fibrosis and cirrhosis. RYGB has shown improved steatosis in three studies [47–49].

Thyroid Disorders

Chronic dieting can result in a significant decrease in intracellular and circulating triiodothyronine (T3) levels [50–52], which drastically reduces basal metabolic rate by 15%–40%. This is an adaptive measure the body takes to conserve energy according to Denis Wilson, MD [53]. Thyroid levels and metabolism stay in a starvation mode making weight loss difficult.

Various studies found that T3 levels were significantly decreased with no difference in thyroid stimulating hormone (TSH) and thyroxine (T4) levels (therefore not able to be detected by routine TSH testing) [54,55]. The reduced T3 may contribute to fatigue and depression expressed by many bariatric surgery candidates. Many of these people have difficulty keeping weight off and are not excessive eaters. Unless the thyroid dysfunction is corrected, weight loss may be far less from the surgery than needed to correct metabolic issues.

Croxson and Ibbertson found that individuals with a history of intense dieting had dramatic reductions in T4 to T3 conversion that led to an intracellular deficiency of T3 that a TSH and T4 test failed to detect [56]. According to Dr. Wilson [53], numerous studies have shown that insulin resistance, diabetes, and metabolic syndrome are associated with reduced T4 to T3 conversion, an intracellular deficiency of T3, and an increased conversion of T4 to reverse T3 (rT3) [57–59].

Hashimoto's thyroiditis (also called chronic lymphocytic thyroiditis) is an autoimmune disorder [60] and is considered the most common cause of thyroid problems in the United States. Hashimoto's disorder is usually diagnosed between the ages of 30 and 50 with more women than men affected, usually as a result of a goiter. Antithyroglobulin antibodies (anti-TG) are elevated in more than 90% of the patients [61] while patients with elevated thyroid peroxidase antibodies (anti-TPO) may be asymptomatic until the disease progresses further.

Nutritional status of bariatric surgery patients can also play a role in hypothyroidism development. Vitamins A, E, B$_{12}$, riboflavin, and niacin deficiency plus inadequate selenium, iodine, iron, zinc, and potassium can alter the metabolism of T4 to T3 in peripheral tissues [62–64]. Excess consumption of goitrogenic foods—cabbage, kale, Brussels sprouts, cauliflower and soy—can induce hypothyroidism.

Since obesity is directly associated with thyrotropin (TSH) and thyroid function, comprehensive thyroid testing needs to be considered since imbalances can affect virtually every metabolic process in the body from mood to energy level. Common symptoms caused from hypothyroidism are

- Fatigue
- Decreased heart rate
- Progressive hearing loss
- Weight gain
- Problems with memory and concentration
- Depression
- Goiter (enlarged thyroid gland)
- Muscle pain or weakness
- Loss of interest in sex
- Numb, tingling hands
- Dry skin
- Swollen eyelids
- Dryness, loss or premature graying of hair
- Extreme sensitivity to cold
- Constipation
- Irregular menstrual periods
- Hoarse voice

A comprehensive thyroid assessment includes: high-sensitivity thyroid stimulating hormone (hTSH), free serum thyroxine (fT4), free triiodothyronine (fT3), rT3, anti-TG, and anti-TPO.

Several studies have been reported about the weight loss after bariatric surgery influencing thyroid hormone regulation possibly through the decreasing leptin influence on peripheral hormone metabolism [65]. Weight loss after RYGB increased free thyroxine (T4) with no change in TSH concentration [66] but Alagna et al. [67] reported decreased fT3 postsurgery and proposed it as a result of reduced peripheral conversion of T4 to fT3.

Subclinical hypothyroidism defined as elevated TSH is consistent in some morbidly obese patients and resolves after bariatric surgery [68,69]. Fazylov studied 20 morbidly obese females who underwent RYGB while on thyroid replacement therapy and found 5 of the 20 had worsened hypothyroidism postsurgery. These cases were identified as having thyroid autoimmune disease [70].

Absorption of levothyroxine, used for the treatment of hypothyroidism, is affected by many factors. The pharmacokinetics in Gkotsina's review of thyroid replacement absorption indicates that the stomach, duodenum, and upper part of the jejunum are not sites of T4 uptake because RYGB and SLG patients had no alteration in absorption postsurgery [71].

A liquid formulation for treatment of hypothyroidism postbariatric surgery is available [72] but Michalaki et al. report that iodine, which is essential for the synthesis of thyroid hormones, should be considered for supplementation [73] in addition.

Sleeve gastrectomy evaluation on patients with normal thyroid function presurgery indicated a decrease in TSH and steady levels of fT4 during their weight loss [74].

Polycystic Ovary Syndrome

PCOS is one of the most common causes of infertility due to anovulation, which leads to obesity from hyperandrogenism and insulin-resistance or metabolic syndrome [75]. Some studies have found a higher incidence of PCOS among women with type 1 and type 2 diabetes. Many times the condition is misdiagnosed or overlooked.

PCOS occurs when excessive male hormone is produced in the ovaries, throwing off the balance of hormones that causes a regular menstrual cycle. Common symptoms are weight gain, acne, and hair growth on the face, chest, and abdomen. The cause of PCOS is unknown but family history may be involved.

PCOS, also known as Stein–Leventhal syndrome, is an endocrine disorder that affects how a woman's ovaries function. Cysts develop on the ovaries and the ovary does not regularly release eggs while hyperandrogenism, or excess male hormone, disrupts the normal ovulation process [76]. Adolescent and young women who have irregular menstrual cycles and do not ovulate are inclined to gain weight and should be assessed for PCOS. Since there is no cure, medication and lifestyle changes can begin early to offset weight problems.

PCOS affects 5%–10% women of reproductive age and up to 50% of them become diabetic or prediabetic before they reach the age of 40 [76]. Dr. Evanthia Diamanti-Kandarakis, Endrocrine Section First Department of Medicine, Medical School, University of Athens, Greece says women with PCOS may have beta cells already prone to dysfunction and insulin resistance just aggravates the problem [76].

Many women with PCOS have had a weight problem their entire life while others indicate it was a sudden onset. Metformin has become a treatment of choice since it may enhance tissue sensitivity to insulin. The effectiveness of metformin rests in its capacity to suppress glucose production by the liver and decrease insulin resistance in the muscle [77].

Metabolic disturbances are common in women with PCOS and obesity is the major link with diabetes, hypertension, and low-grade inflammation. Preventative measures of diet, exercise, and smoking cessation for weight loss are difficult to achieve with hormonal imbalance so bariatric surgery can reduce risks of morbid obesity in PCOS [78–80]. PCOS is also associated with insulin resistance and metabolic syndrome according to Caserta et al. [81] and it is necessary to treat excess adiposity and the insulin resistance in order to prevent cardiovascular disease.

Gastric bypass surgery achieved significant reduction in BMI, testosterone, blood glucose, and lipid metabolism in PCOS cases [82] and sleeve gastrectomy resolved endocrine mechanisms in a woman who did not respond to insulin sensitizing drugs for treatment of her PCOS [83].

A meta-analysis of 13 studies involving 2,130 female patients with PCOS has shown bariatric surgery to be a successful management strategy for morbid obesity but limited data exists on the effectiveness in symptom management of PCOS [84]. Barber and Dimitriadis [85] make the association of PCOS with obesity based on genetic studies and suggest dietary modifications and exercise are important in weight loss maintenance.

Improved eating behavior for management of clinical symptoms of PCOS is stressed in two studies reviewing the need for lifestyle modification to improve success in not only weight loss but fertility and hormone levels [86,87]. Using a low-glycemic diet is important for symptom management.

MTHFR Polymorphisms

The Human Genome Project and the subsequent identification of single nucleotide polymorphisms (SNPs) have led to the concept of personalized medicine and personalized nutrition therapy or nutrigenomics [88]. Polymorphisms have been slow to catch on in medical practice but the *MTHFR* genes can be assessed by most diagnostic laboratories.

The *MTHFR* gene testing is a way of detecting the efficiency of the methylation cycle that occurs in each cell of the body to carry out energy production, detoxification, immune function, inflammation management, and gene replication [89]. Methylation defects contribute to addictions, chronic infections, anxiety, cardiovascular disease, diabetes, fibromyalgia, infertility, irritable bowel syndrome, migraines, neural tube defects, rheumatoid arthritis, sleep disorders, stroke, thyroid dysfunction, and many other medical conditions that a bariatric patient can present with. An estimated 30% of the population may have methylation defect genetic markers where they do not make the enzyme for methylfolate production [90]. The *MTHFR* gene provides instructions for making an enzyme called MTHFR along with playing a vital role in processing amino acids. A deficiency of the enzyme can be identified when homocysteine is elevated because it cannot be converted to methionine.

Both *MTHFR* mutations C677T and A1298C cannot convert folic acid into folate, which is needed for proper methylation. Conditions related to these *MTHFR* defects are: miscarriages, chronic pain, insomnia, fibromyalgia, neurological disorders, neural tube defects, elevated histamine, cardiovascular risk, hypertension, depression, cleft palate, autism, headaches/migraines, IBS, chronic fatigue, chemical sensitivity, thyroid dysfunction, anxiety, bipolar disorder, infertility, multiple sclerosis, addictive behaviors, and allergies [90].

- Conditions common with C677T: elevated homocysteine, cardiovascular disease, stroke, peripheral neuropathy, neural tube defects, cleft palate, blood clots, stillbirths, deep vein thrombosis

- Conditions common with A1298C: depression, anxiety, IBS, fibromyalgia, chronic fatigue, dementia, schizophrenia, Parkinson's, migraines

Little is known about SNPs and overweight/obesity but Yin et al. [91,92] reported several polymorphisms that included those in *MTHFR*, influencing overweight/obesity. Another study on four population groups in the United Kingdom and Denmark found the *MTHFR* C677T genotype to be associated with an increased risk of obesity BMI>30 [93]. A Saudi study confirmed that the genetic polymorphisms *MTHFR* C677T and A1298C are associated with the risk of hypertension in patients with obesity and diabetes [94]. Koo et al. found the MTHFR association with homocysteine predictive of the development of premature coronary heart disease in hypertensive adolescents [95].

The *MTHFR* polymorphisms are associated with various diseases—vascular, cancer, neurology, diabetes, psoriasis, and so forth. Homozygous mutated patients have higher homocysteine levels, which usually need supplementation with vitamin B_{12} and folate [96]. Lunegova et al. reported this same *MTHFR* allele was associated with insulin resistance, abdominal obesity and hypertriglyceridemia [97]. Other studies confirmed the association of *MTHFR* C677T genotype in diabetes, insulin resistance, and obesity [97,98].

MTHFR genetic mutation testing is becoming a useful tool in nutrition assessment for personalizing dietary recommendations [99, 100]. Since bariatric surgery is rapidly becoming the treatment of choice for obesity, nutrition management needs to consider all aspects of the malabsorption caused by the surgery and genetic factors that may contribute. An example of how nutrigenomics needs to quickly evolve is provided by Yarandi et al. They present a case of an undiagnosed copper deficiency postgastric bypass where a heterozygous *MTHFR* A1298C gene polymorphism resulted in irreversible neurological manifestations even after copper repletion [101].

Overcoming the *MTHFR* defects usually requires adequate folate, a critical cofactor in metabolism. Mammals cannot synthesize folate and depend on food sources and/or supplementation to maintain normal levels [102]. Low-folate levels may be caused from poor food choices, poor absorption of the ingested folate, or drug–nutrient interactions. Supplementation of folic acid or fortified foods instead of the recommended 5-MTHFR can lead to negative effects of unconverted folic acid in peripheral circulation [102]. Preventing folate deficiency in patients with *MTHFR* polymorphisms is imperative to their health.

Food Sources of Folate

Green leafy vegetables are rich sources of folate, providing the basis for its name. Citrus fruits and legumes are also excellent sources.

Leaf lettuce 1 cup	40 µg
Kale, chopped 1 cup	19 µg
Spinach, cooked 1 cup	263 µg
Orange, raw 1	47 µg
Chickpeas, cooked 1/2 cup	141 µg

CASE STUDIES

Polycystic Ovary Syndrome

BC, a 43-year-old female 7 years postlapband surgery, considers gastric bypass since her band has slipped resulting in dysphagia and reflux. She was initially successful in weight loss after lap-band placement but currently weighs 305 lb., BMI: 47.8, body fat: 52.5%. She had previously been prescribed metformin but currently does not take it.

24-hour food intake: Breakfast: not eaten regularly, sometimes protein drink; Lunch: turkey patty, chips and salsa; Snack: yogurt or bagel and coffee; Dinner: ice cream or cereal then off to bed.

Labs drawn included complete blood count (CBC), comprehensive metabolic panel (CMP), thyroid, vitamin D, *MTHFR*, prolactin, sex hormone-binding globulin (SHBG), high-sensitivity C-reactive protein (hs-CRP), progesterone, estradiol. Results indicate no *MTHFR* variant, hs-CRP: 9.5, A1c: 5.6%, TSH: 1.44, thyroid antibodies: 0, vitamin D_3: 58.

BC is unable to lose weight on high-protein low-carbohydrate diet 7 days postnutrition counseling. Discussion focused on importance of regular eating schedule—especially breakfast to control blood glucose. One month after nutrition consult prior to scheduling gastric bypass surgery, weight: 302 lb., labs indicate hs-CRP: 8.6, antinuclear antibody (ANA) negative. Viral load: Epstein–Barr virus (EBV), Cytomegalovirus (CMV), *Mycoplasma pneumoniae*, *Yersinia*. Oral antiviral treatment commenced, while patient considering antiviral IV treatment. Patient fears she would not be able to lose weight after gastric bypass.

Polycystic Ovary Syndrome

JS, a 36-year-old female weighing 206 lb., BMI: 35.4, body fat: 41.7%, reports being overweight since age 13. The roller coaster weight loss associates with a diagnosis of Hashimoto's thyroiditis (Synthroid), depression (lexapro), PCOS (aldactone) with metformin recommended for elevated testosterone.

24-hour food intake: Breakfast: melon + protein bar; Lunch: salad or sandwich; Dinner: "anything" like beef with pasta and vegetable. Denies snacking due to exhaustion and goes straight to bed.

Nutrition counseling provided menu guide pre- and post-surgery for ketogenic low-carbohydrate diet for better thyroid and energy management. She reports being too tired to exercise.

Hypothyroid

SH, a 54-year-old female 4 years postlapband, is "always hungry." She has been prescribed Synthroid for 3 years. Current weight: 275 lb., BMI: 39.6, body fat: 51%.

24-hour food recall: Breakfast: (eaten at desk) oatmeal with raisins, banana, coffee; Snack: Kashi bar and fruit; Lunch: turkey sandwich and beans; Dinner: beans and beef brisket; Snack: cake and ice cream.

Nutrition counseling advised her to follow ketogenic diet to try and control hunger. She needs to discuss changing her thyroid medication with her primary physician.

(*continued*)

Gastric Bypass Surgery Complications

TL is a 48-year-old female with prior knee and hysterectomy surgeries, *H. pylori* and fatty liver issues + thyroid ablation for nodule 10 years prior. Currently suffers from migraines treated with medication. Weight: 223.6 lb., BMI: 38.4, body fat: 44.9%. She reports her weight at 18 was 127 lb.

24-hour food intake: sometimes yogurt or breakfast sandwich; Lunch: bacon, lettuce, and tomato (BLT) or salad (office delivery); Dinner: (11 PM or midnight) sandwich or drive-thru.

Two months postgastric bypass surgery patient arrives stating 2-day surgery turned into 5-day hospitalization + blood transfusion + UTI. Weight: 184.6 lb., BMI: 31.7, body fat 40.6%. She had stopped losing weight in the past 2 weeks. Labs were drawn to assess metabolic function. Patient reports she had weekly B_{12} shots 10 years prior to help migraines.

Current postsurgery diet: Breakfast: 1/2 cup black coffee; Lunch: tuna or chicken salad (1/4 cup); Snack: sugar-free gelatin; Dinner: 3 oz. chicken + steamed vegetables.

One week later: no change in weight, BMI, and body fat. Labs reviewed: Cholesterol: 264, triglycerides: 213, blood glucose: 105, AST/ALT: within normal limits (wnl), albumin (Alb): 4.1, hs-CRP: 10.2, vitamin D: 37, A1c: 4.9%, folate: 8.3, vitamin B_{12}: 736, red blood cell distribution width (RDW): 15.6% (H), TSH: 1.13, fT3: 3.31, fT4: 1.08, *MTHFR*: AC heterozygous.

Nutrition Plan of Care: 50,000 IM 25-OH vitamin D, methylcobalamin and B complex IM every other day with reassessment in 30 days. Discuss elevated hs-CRP with primary care physician due to inflammation/infection. Continue ketogenic diet for weight loss.

MTHFR *and Repeat Gastric Bypass*

RM is a 49-year-old female hypothyroid, on Synthroid, posthysterectomy and had gastric bypass 6 years prior. Current weight: 271.6 lb., BMI: 43.2, body fat: 51.3%.

24-hour food recall: Breakfast: not regularly eaten or protein shake; Lunch: leftovers or sandwich and grapes; Dinner: chicken and vegetables; Snack: homemade snack balls or fruit.

Labs: Blood glucose: 86, ANA: negative, *MTHFR*: AC homozygous, TSH: 3.5, T3: 64 (L), TPO: 157 (H), thyroid antibodies: 9.9 (H), vitamin D: 39.2, hs-CRP: 5.28 (H).

Patient hopes repeat gastric bypass will reduce risk of cardiovascular issues. Nutrition counseling stressed need for ketogenic diet for weight loss and increased exercise. Reviewed guidelines for MTHFR deficiency and nutrition but patient prefers to get surgery done before further changes are made.

Prediabetes

SS is a 54-year-old, prediabetic female with hypertension × 15 years and family history of thyroid goiter problems. Rx: pramipexole and fluoxetine. Reports vitamin D deficient × 6 years. Weight: 304.6 lb., BMI: 47.7, body fat: 53.4%.

24-Hour food recall: "Knows she eats too much" Breakfast: Organic cereal, almond milk, banana + walnuts; Lunch: 1/2 peanut butter sandwich on whole wheat; Dinner: salmon, yellow rice, broccoli; Snack: yogurt.

Labs: Cholesterol: 234, T: 195, BG: 129, hs-CRP: 5.8, vitamin D: 26, *MTHFR*: CT heterozygous, A1c: 6.1, Insulin: 82.6, vitamin B_{12}: 403, folate: 12.6, TSH: 1.03, fT3 3.88, thyroid antibodies: 31.2 (H), ferritin: 250 (H). Provided vitamin D and B_{12} IM postlab draw.

Lab review with patient—she reports feeling better after B_{12} and vitamin D in the past week and states ferritin has been high for several years. Menu plans for ketogenic diet provided and advised to discuss labs with primary care physician.

Type 1 Diabetes

CM is a 32-year-old female with diabetes on sliding scale humalog + lantus HS 2 weeks postgastric bypass. She has lost 28 lb. but cannot lose any more despite calorie and carbohydrate counting. She stated that the physician told her diabetes would be resolved postsurgery. Weight 247.4 lb., BMI: 41, body fat 48.6%.

24-hour food recall: protein drink × 2, chili, 1/2 banana, 4 oz. juice, lean cuisine, 6 grapes. (Blood glucose: 81–235 monitored at each food intake—.) Provided daily log × 3 days with BG: 107–255.

(continued)

Labs: BG (nonfasting): 290, TSH: 1.22, *MTHFR*: AC het-erozygous, hs-CRP: 4.1 (H).

Nutrition consult and lab review advising continued keto-genic diet. She states she does not feel or look different since her surgery. Reviewed diabetes management for Type 1 insulin dependent individuals but she was very overwhelmed that she would continue to need insulin.

References

1. Plaisted CS, Istfan NW. *Metabolic abnormalities of obesity. Obesity Pathophysiology Psychology and Treatment.* In: Blackburn GL, Kanders BS, eds. New York, NY: Chapman & Hall 1994.
2. Tailleux A, Rouskas K, Pattou F, et al. Bariatric surgery, lipoprotein metabolism and cardiovascular risk. *Curr Opin Lipidol* 2015;26:317–324.
3. Kaplan NH. Hypertension and hyperinsulinemia. *Prim Care* 1991;18:483.
4. Reaven GM. Banting Lecture 1988. Role of insulin resistance in human disease. *Diabetes* 37:1595.
5. Feingold KR, Grunfeld C. Obesity and dyslipidemia. In: De Groot LJ, Beck-Peccoz P, Chrousos G, et al., eds. *Endotext* [Internet]. South Dartmouth, MA: MDText.com, Inc.; 2000. Available at: http://www .ncbi.nlm.nih.gov/books/NBK305895/.
6. Padilla N, Maraninchi M, Béliard S, et al. Effects of bariatric surgery on hepatic and intestinal lipoprotein particle metabolism in obese, non-diabetic humans. *Arterioscler Thromb Vasc Biol* 2014;34:2330–2337.
7. Batsis JA, Miranda WR, Prasad C, et al. Effect of bariatric surgery on cardiovascular risk in elderly patients: A population-based study. *Geriatr Gerontol Int* 2015;16:618–624.
8. Domienik-Karlowicz J, Dzikowska-Diduch O, Lisik W, et al. Short-term cardiometabolic risk reduction after bariatric surgery. *Hellanic J Cardiol* 2015;56:61–65.
9. Corcellas R, Daigle CR, Schauer PR. Management of endocrine diseases: Metabolic effects of bariatric surgery. *Eur J Endocrinol* 2016;174:R19–28.
10. Morshed G, Fathy SM. Impact of post-laparoscopic sleeve gastrectomy weight loss on C-reactive protein, lipid profile and CA-125 in morbidly obese women. *Wideochir Inne Tech Maloinwazyjne* 2016;10:521–526.
11. McLellan KCP, Wyne K, Villagomez ET, et al. Pharmacologic treatment of prediabetes. *Pract Diabetel.* 2014 May/June;33:6–11.
12. Bell DSH. Metformin: A lifesaver for those with and without diabetes. *Practical Diabetology.* 2016 March/April;35:16–17.
13. Guilliford MC, Booth HP, Reddy M, et al. Effect of contemporary bariatric surgery procedures on Type 2 diabetes remission—A population-based matched cohort study. *Obes Surg* 2016 Feb 27. [Epub ahead of print.]

14. Omotosho P, Mor A, Shantavasinkul PC, et al. Gastric bypass significantly improves quality of life in morbidly obese patients with type 2 diabetes. *Surg Endosc* 2016;28. [Epub ahead of print.]
15. deOliveira LF, Tisott CG, Silvano DM, et al. Glycemic behavior in 48 hours postoperative period of patients with type 2 diabetes mellitus and nondiabetic submitted to bariatric surgery. *Arg Bras Cir Dig* 2015;28:26–30.
16. Hansen M, Lund MT, Jørgensen AL, et al. The effects of diet-and RYGB-induced weight loss on insulin sensitivity in obese oatients with and without Type 2 diabetes. *Acta Diabetol* 2015;53:423–432.
17. Yaska JP, vanRoon EN, de Boer A, et al. Remission of Type 2 diabetes mellitus in patients after different types of bariatric surgery: A population-based cohort study in the United Kingdom. *JAMA Surgery* 2015 Dec 1;150(12):1126–1133.
18. Pappachan JM, Viswanath AK. Metabolic surgery: A paradigm shift in Type 2 diabetes management. *World J Diabetes* 2015 Dec 1;150(12)1126–1133.
19. Warren JA, Ewing JA, Hale AL, et al. Cost-effectiveness of bariatric surgery: Increasing the economic viability of the most effective treatment for Type II Diabetes Mellitus. *Am Surg* 2015;81:807–811.
20. Argyropoulos G. Bariatric surgery: Prevalence, predictors, and mechanisms of diabetes remission. *Curr Diab Rep* 2015;15:15.
21. Cummings DE. Surgery to treat diabetes vs lifestyle interventions. *Obesity Week* 2013.
22. Fanin A, Benetti A, Ceriani V, et al. Bariatric surgery versus medications in the treatment of Type 2 diabetes. *Minerva Endocrinol* 2015;40:297–306.
23. Hsu CC, Almulaifi A, Chen JC, et al. Effect of bariatric surgery vs medical treatment on Type 2 diabetes on patients with body mass index lower than 35: Five-year outcomes. *JAMA Surgery* 2015 Dec 1;150(12):1117–1124.
24. Singh AK, Singh R, Kota SK. Bariatric surgery and diabetes remission: Who would have thought it? *Indian J Endocrinol Metab* 2015 Sept–Oct;19(5):563–576.
25. Chen Y, Corsino L, Shantavasinkul PC, et al. Gastric bypass leads to long-term remission or improvement of type 2 diabetes and significant decrease of microvascular and macrovascular complications. *Ann Surg* 2016;263(6):1138–1142.
26. Brethauer SA, Aminian A, Romero-Talamás H, et al. Can diabetes be surgically cured? Long-term metabolic effects of bariatric surgery in obese patients with Type 2 diabetes mellitus. *Ann Surg* 2013;258: 628–637.
27. Panunji S, Carlsson L, De Gaetano A, et al. Determinants of diabetes remission and glycemic control after bariatric surgery. *Diabetes Care* 2016;39:166–174.
28. Grams J, Garvey WT. Weight loss and the prevention and treatment of Type 2 diabetes using lifestyle therapy, pharmacotherapy and bariatric surgery: Mechanisms of action. *Curr Obes Rep* 2015;4:287–302.

29. Cefalu WT, Bray GA, Home PD, et al. Advances in the science, treatment and prevention of the disease of obesity: Reflections form a diabetes care editors' expert forum. *Diabetes Care* 2015;38:1567–1582.

30. Khanna V, Malin SK, Bena J, et al. Adults with long-duration Type 2 diabetes have blunted glycemic and B cell function improvement after bariatric surgery. *Obesity* 2015;23:523–256.

31. Jukubowicz D, Wainstein J, Ahren B, et al. Fasting until noon triggers increased postprandial hyperglycemia and impaired insulin response after lunch and dinner in individuals with Type 2 diabetes: A randomized clinical trial. *Diabetes Care* 2015;38:1820–1826.

32. Seaman AM. Bariatric surgery edges out lifestyle changes for Type 2 diabetes. *JAMA Surgery* 2015.

33. Courcoulas AP, Belle BH, Neiberg RH, et al. Three year outcomes of bariatric surgery vs lifestyle intervention for Type 2 diabetes mellitus treatment. *JAMA Surgery* 2015;150:931–940.

34. Dogan K, Betzel B, Homan J, et al. Long-term effects of laparoscopic Roux-en-Y gastric bypass on diabetes mellitus, hypertension and dyslipidemia in morbidly obese patients. *Obes Surg* 2014;24:1835–1842.

35. Xiong SW, Cao J, Liu XM, et al. Effect of modified Roux-en-Y gastric bypass surgery on GLP-1, GIP in patients with Type 2 diabetes mellitus. *Gastroenterol Res Pract* 2015;62:5196.

36. Golomb J, Bendavid M, Glass A, et al. Long-term metabolic effects of laparoscopic sleeve gastrectomy. *JAMA Surgery* 2015;150:1051–1057.

37. Ashrafian H, Harling L, Toma T, et al. Type 1 diabetes mellitus and bariatric surgery: A systemic review and meta-analysis. *Obes Surg* 2015 Dec 22.

38. Mahawar KK, De Alwis N, Carr WR, et al. Bariatric surgery in Type 1 diabetes mellitus: A systemic review. *Obes Surg* 2016;26:196–204.

39. Markova M et al. Better blood glucose control found with high-protein diets from plant, animal sources. *Endocrine Today*, Nov 2015.

40. Martínez-González MA, de la Fuente-Arrillaga C, Nunez-Cordoba JM, et al. Adherence to Mediterranean diet and risk of developing diabetes: Prospective cohort study. *BMJ* 2005;336:1348–1351.

41. Lacoppidan SA, Kyrø C, Loft S, et al. Adherence to a healthy nordic food index is associated with lower risk of Type 2 diabetes—The Danish Diet, Cancer and Health Cohort Study. *Nutrients* 2015;7:8633–8644.

42. Saudi J. The effect of bariatric surgeries on nonalcoholic fatty liver disease. *Gastroenterol* 2014 Sept–Oct; 20(5): 270–278.

43. Clark JM, Alkhuraishi AR, Solga SF, et al. Roux-en-Y gastric bypass improves liver histology in patients with non-alcoholic fatty liver disease. *Obes Res* 2005;13:1180–1186.

44. Feijó SG, Lima JM, Oliveira MA, et al. The spectrum of non alcoholic fatty liver disease in morbidly obese patients: Prevalence and associated risk factors. *Acta Cir Bras* 2013;28:788–793.

45. Xanthakos SA, Jenkins TM, Kleiner DE, et al. High prevalence of non alcoholic fatty liver disease in adolescents undergoing bariatric surgery. *Gastroenterology* 2015;149:623–634.

46. Sasaki A, Nitta H, Otsuka K, et al. Bariatric surgery and non-alcoholic fatty liver disease: Current and potential future treatments. *Front Endocrinol* 2014;27:164.
47. Weiner RA. Surgical treatment of non-alcoholic steatohepatitis and non-alcoholic fatty liver disease. *Dig Dis* 2010;28:274–279.
48. deAlmeida SR, Rocha PR, Sanches MD, et al. Roux-en-Y bypass improves the nonalcoholic steatohepatitis (NASH) of morbid obesity. *Obes Surg* 2006;16:270–278.
49. Liu X, Lazenby AJ, Clements RH, et al. Resolution of non-alcoholic steatohepatitis after gastric bypass surgery. *Obes Surg* 2007;17:486–492.
50. Cheron RG, Kaplan MM, Larsen PR. Physiological and pharmacological influences on thyroxine to 3,5,3-triiodothyronine conversion and nuclear 3,5,3-triiodothyronine binding in rat anterior pituitary. *J Clin Invest* 1979;64:1402–1414.
51. Araujo RL, Andrade BM, da Silva ML, et al. Tissue specific deiodinase regulation during food restriction and low replacement dose of leptin in rats. *Am J Physiol Endocrinol Metab* 2009;296:E1157–1163.
52. Leibel RL, Jirsch J. Diminished energy requirements in reduced-obese patients. *Metabolism* 1984;33:164–170.
53. Wilson D. *Evidence-Based Approach to Restoring Thyroid Health*. Lady Lake, FL: Muskeegee Medical Publishing, 2014.
54. Fontana L, Klein S, Holloszy JO, et al. Effect of long-term calorie restriction with adequate protein and micronutrients on thyroid hormones. *J Clin Endocrinol Metab* 2006;91:3232–3235.
55. Silva JE, Larsen PR. Hormonal regulation iodothyronine 5'-deiodinase in rat brown adipose tissue. *Am J Physiol* 251;E639–E643.
56. Croxson MS, Ibbertson HK. Low serum triiodothyronine (T3) and hypothyroidism. *J Clin Endocrinol Metab* 1977;44:167–174.
57. Katzeff HL, Selgrad C. Impaired peripheral thyroid hormone metabolism in genetic obesity. *Endocrinology* 1993;132:989–995.
58. Islam S., Yesmire S, Khan SA, et al. A comparative study of thyroid hormone levels in diabetic and non-diabetic patients. *SE Asian J Trop Med Public Health* 2008;39:913–916.
59. Benvenga S, Cahnmann HJ, Robbins J. Characterization of thyroid hormone binding to apolipoprotein E: Localization of the binding site in the exon 3-coded domain. *Endocrinology* 1993;133:1300–1305.
60. McLeod DS, Cooper DS. The incidence and prevalence of thyroid auto-immunity. *Endocrine* 2012;42:252–265.
61. McGrogan A, Seaman HE, Wright JW, et al. The incidence of auto-immune thyroid disease: A systematic review of the literature. *Clin Endocrinol* 2008;69:687–696.
62. Delange F. The disorders induced by iodine deficiency. *Thyroid* 1994;4:107–128.
63. Pizzulli A, Ranjbar A. Selenium deficiency and hypothyroidism: A new etiology in the differential diagnosis of hypothyroidism in children. *Biol Trace Elem Res* 2000;77:199–208.

64. Watts DL. The nutritional relationship of the thyroid. *J Orthomol Med* 1989;4:165–169.
65. Lips MA, Pyl H, van Klinken JB, et al. Roux-en-Y gastric bypass and calorie restriction induce comparable time-dependent effects on thyroid hormone function tests in obese female subjects. *Eur J Endocrinol* 2013 Aug 28;169(3):339–347.
66. MacCuish A, Razvi S, Syed AA. Effect of weight loss after gastric bypass surgery on thyroid function in euthyroid people with morbid obesity. *Clin Obes* 2012 Feb;2(1–2):25–28.
67. Alagna S, Cossu ML, Masala A, et al. Evaluation of serum leptin levels and thyroid function in morbidly obese patients treated with bariatric surgery. *Eat Weight Dis* 2003 Jun;8(2):95–99.
68. Janssen IM, Homan J, Schijns W, et al. Subclinical hypothyroidism and its relation to obesity in patients before and after Roux-en Y gastric bypass. *Surg Obes Relat Dis* 2015 Nov–Dec;11(6):1257–63.
69. Chikunguwo S, Brethauer S, Nirujogi V, et al. Influence of obesity and surgical weight loss on thyroid hormone levels. *Surg Obes Relat Dis* 2007 Nov–Dec;3(6):631–35.
70. Fazylov R, Soto E, Cohen S, et al. Laaparoscopic Roux-en-Y gastric bypass surgery on morbidly obese patients with hypothyroidism. *Obes Surg* 2008 Jun;18(6):644–647.
71. Gkotsina M, Michalaki M, Mamali I, et al. Improved levothroxine pharmacokinetics after bariatric surgery. *Thyroid* 2013 Apr; 23(4):414–419.
72. Vita R, Fallahi P, Antonelli A, et al. The administration of thyroxine as a soft gel capsule or liquid solution. *Expert Opin Drug Deliv* 2014 Jul; 11(7):1103–1111.
73. Michalaki M, Volonakis S, Mamali I, et al. Dietary iodine absorption is not influenced by malabsorptive bariatric surgery. *Obes Surg* 2014 Nov;24(11):1921–1925.
74. Abu-Ghanem Y, Inbar R, Tyomkin V, et al. Effect of sleeve gastrectomy on thyroid hormone levels. *Obes Surg* 2015 Mar;25(3):452–456.
75. Dunaif A, Chang J, Franks S, et al eds. In: *Contemporary Endocrinology*. Totowa, NJ: Humana Press, 2008, p. 217.
76. Davies N. Polycystic ovary syndrome. *Diabetes Self Management* Feb 2016.
77. Thatcher SS. *PCOS the Hidden Epidemic*. Indianapolis, IN: Perspectives Press, 2000, p. 156.
78. Escobar-Morreale HF. Surgical management of metabolic dysfunction in PCOS. *Steroids* 2012 Mar 10;77(4):312–316.
79. Ollila MM, Piltonen T, Puukka, et al. Weight gain and dyslipidemia in early adulthood associate with polycystic ovary syndrome: Prospective cohort study. *J Clin Endocrinol Metab* 2016;101:739–747.
80. Messinis IE, Messini CI, Anifandis G, et al. Polycystic ovaries and obesity. *Best Pract Res Clin Obstet Gynaecol* 2015 May;29(4):479–488.
81. Caserta D, Adducchio G, Picchia S, et al. Metabolic syndrome and polycystic ovary syndrome: An intriguing relationship. *Gynecol Endocrinol* 2014 Jun;30(6):397–402.

82. Eid GM, McCloskey C, Titchner R, et al. Changes in hormones and biomarkers in polycystic ovarian syndrome treated with gastric bypass. *Surg Obes Relat Dis* 2014 Sept–Oct;10(5):787–791.

83. Schiavo L, Scalera G, Barbarisi A. Sleeve gastrectomy to treat concommitant polycystic ovary syndrome, insulin and leptin resistance in a 27-year morbidly obese woman unresponsive to insulin-sensitizing drugs: A 3-year follow-up. *Int J Surg Case Rep* 2015 Oct 21;17:36–38.

84. Skubleny D, Switzer NJ, Gill RS, et al. The impact of bariatric surgery on polycystic ovary syndrome: A systematic review and meta-analysis. *Obes Surg* 2016 Jan;26(1):169–176.

85. Barber TM, Dimitriadis GK, Andreou A, et al. Polycystic ovary syndrome: Insight into pathogenesis and a common association with insulin resistance. *Clin Med (Lond)* 2015 Dec;15(Suppl 6):S72–S76.

86. Turkmen S, Andreen L, Cengiz Y. Effects of Roux-en-Y gastric bypass surgery on eating behavior and allopregnanolone levels in obese women with polycystic ovary syndrome. *Gynecol Endocrinol* 2015 Apr;31(4):301–305.

87. Moran LJ, Brinkworth GD, Norman RJ. Dietary therapy in polycystic ovary syndrome. *Semin Reprod Med* 2008 Jan;26:85–92.

88. Subbiah MT. Nutrigenetics and nutraceuticals: The next wave riding on personalized medicine. *Transl Res* 2007 Feb;149(2):55–61.

89. Frankel F. *The Methylation Miracle*. New York, NY: St. Martin's Press, 1999.

90. Miller R, Bowers B. *MethylGenetic Nutrition Breaking the Genetic Code*. Philadelphia, PA, Nov 7–8, 2015.

91. Yin RX, Wu DF, Aung LH, et al. Several lipid-related gene polymorphisms interact with overweight/obesity to moderate blood pressure levels. *Int J Mol Sci* 2012;13(9):2062–2081.

92. Yin RX, Wu DF, Miao L, et al. Several genetic polymorphisms interact with overweight/obesity in influence serum lipid levels. *Cardiovasc Diabetol* 2012 Oct 8; 11:123.

93. Lewis SJ, Lawlor DA, Nordestgaard BG, et al. The methylenetetrahydrofolate reductase C677T genotype and the risk of obesity in three large population-based cohorts. *Eur J Endocrinol* 2008 Jul;159(1):35–40.

94. Alghasham A, Settin AA, Ali A, et al. Association of MTHFR C677T and A1298C gene polymorphisms with hypertension. *Int J Health Sci* 2012 Jan;6(1):3–11.

95. Koo HS, Lee HS, Hong YM. Methylenetetrahydrofolate reductase TT genotype as a predictor of cardiovascular risk in hypertensive adolescents. *Pediatr Cardiol* 2008 Jan;29(1):136–141.

96. Liew SC, Gupta ED. Methylenetetrahydrofolate reductase (MTHFR) C677T polymorphism: Epidemiology, metabolism and associated diseases. *Eur J Med Genet* 2015 Jan;58(1):1–10.

97. Lunegova OS, Kerimkulova AS, Turdakmatov NB, et al. Association of C677T gene polymorphism of methylenetetrahydrofolate reductase with insulin resistance among Kirghizes. *Kardiologiia* 2011;51:58–62.

98. Tavakkoly Bazzaz J, Shojapoor M, et al. Methlenetetrahydrofolate reductase gene polymorphism in diabetes and obesity. *Mol Biol Rep* 2010 Jan;37(1):105–109.

99. Frelut ML, Nicolas JP, Guilland JC, et al. Methylenetetrahydrofolate reductase 677 C→T polymorphism: A link between birth weight and insulin resistance in obese adolescents. *Int J Pediatr Obes.* 2011;6:e312–e317.

100. DiRenzo L, Marsella LT, Sarlo F, et al. C677T gene polymorphism of MTHFR and metabolic syndrome: Response to dietary intervention. *J Transl Med* 2014 Nov 29;12:329.

101. Yarandi SS, Griffith DP, Sharma R, et al. Optic neuropathy, myelopathy, anemia, and neutropenia casued by acquired copper deficiency after gastric bypass surgery. *J Clin Gastroenterol* 2014 Nov–Dec;48(10):862–865.

102. Scaglione F, Panzavolta G. Folate, folic acid and 5-methyltetrahydrofolate are not the same thing. *Xenobiotica* 2014 May;44(5):480–8.

9

PREGNANCY AFTER BARIATRIC SURGERY

Little is known about the impact of bariatric surgery weight loss on pregnancy rate but a meta-analysis of data from 589 infertile obese women indicates a 58% pregnancy rate after surgery [1]. An obesity–fertility protocol study suggests that even a loss of 5%–10% body weight can restore ovulation [2] so contraceptive counseling needs to be considered for women of child bearing age. Pregnancy after bariatric surgery has complications in nutritional and gastrointestinal tract issues that need management by a multidisciplinary team that includes a nutritionist, obstetrician, anesthesiologist along with the bariatric surgeon [3].

Every pregnant woman needs an individual assessment of her nutritional status to identify preconception nutrition issues, medical history, previous reproductive performance, and economic status. Nutritional risk factors during the pregnancy of a bariatric surgery patient need to be outlined especially regarding adequate weight gain and anemia management.

During pregnancy, plasma proteins are diluted so serum albumin of 3.0 g/mL and a total protein value of 6.0 g/mL are considered normal. Blood glucose and glycohemoglobin levels should be monitored regularly to assess gestational diabetes [4]. Anemia is the most common nutritional complication of pregnancy but minimum reports have been published on bariatric surgery cases with respect to this condition.

Gastric bypass surgery increases the risk of gastrointestinal complications during pregnancy with symptoms varying from abdominal pain to nausea and vomiting resulting from internal hernias created by the surgery [5]. Pain is usually exacerbated by eating, which adds intraabdominal pressure as the uterus grows and places pressure on the intestines [6]. As the uterus enlarges, the diaphragm is elevated, which reduces lung capacity by 5% and residual volume by 20% [4]. Kidneys increase slightly in length and weight during pregnancy, which increases glomerular filtration rate but may result in preeclampsia and higher excretion rates of glucose, amino acids, and water-soluble vitamins. Changes along the gastrointestinal tract require increased nutrient intake during pregnancy. Motility of the gut and increased levels of progesterone that reduce motilin may lead to gastric emptying time changes or symptoms of gastrointestinal distress [4], especially in bariatric surgery pregnancy cases.

Gastric banding is not a risk-free surgery for pregnancy according to Jacquemyn and Meesters [7]. They report that a 20-week gestational age female reported to the emergency department with severe nausea and vomiting. Imaging studies were not done to avoid harming the fetus but the patient continued vomiting and fetal death was noted at 23 weeks. When symptoms did not resolve postdelivery, a computed tomography (CT) scan demonstrated gastric band slippage over the pylorus resulting in obstruction. Chevrot et al. discuss the complications from band slippage resulting in dysphagia with no fetal loss [8].

Pregnancy after bariatric surgery does reduce the risk of gestational diabetes and excessive fetal growth but an increased risk of small-for-gestational-age infant with an increased risk of mortality [9]. Due to decreased food intake and variable degrees of malabsorption, newborns are at greater risk for neural defects due to folate malnutrition [10]. Other adverse neonatal outcomes caused from maternal nutrient deficiencies are visual complications (vitamin A), intracranial hemorrhage (vitamin K_1 or phylloquinone), neurological and developmental impairment (vitamin B_{12}) [11]. Vitamin A deficiency in pregnancy after Roux-en-Y Gastric Bypass (RYGB) can represent a high-risk situation and oral supplementation is recommended [12].

A multicenter study, including women with restrictive (lapband) or malabsorptive (gastric bypass) surgeries, reports that most nutrients were depleted and declined significantly during pregnancy. Throughout the first trimester, most women took a multivitamin and during the second- and third trimester, the majority took additional supplements to try to normalize low levels of nutrients [13].

Bariatric surgery malabsorption is associated with increased risk of fetal growth [14] but despite the low birth weight has resulted in adequate growth of these children born after the surgery [15].

Counseling Points

- Weight loss can increase fertility.
- Wait at least 12–18 months before pregnancy. [16]
- Monitor nutrient intake **closely.**
- Educate obstetrics and gynecology (OB-GYN) physicians about weight loss surgery.
- Most choose a Cesarean delivery due to expansion of uterus and increased risk of internal herniation [17].

Monitor for gestational diabetes and pregnancy-induced hypertension Nutrition counseling regime for bariatric pregnancy includes four sessions with a nutritionist to discuss adequate nutrient supplementation, lactation, and pregnancy diet.

Session 1 [6–8 weeks]	Healthy eating, dietary supplements for first trimester
	Physical activity, nausea issues
Session 2 [16–20 weeks]	Body changes/discomforts, dietary supplements and
	increased protein + fatty acid needs
	Screen for gestational diabetes
Session 3 [24–28 weeks]	Assess nutrient status: macro and micronutrients
	Adequate Vitamin D_3, B_{12}, folate
	Preterm labor issues
Session 4 [30–32 weeks]	Diet adequacy for delivery and infant care
	Nutrient supplementation post-pregnancy—especially for lactation

Key Nutrient Needs during Pregnancy

Protein is the major structural component of all cells, and during pregnancy whole body turnover increases as the fetus, uterus, placenta, blood volume, amniotic fluid, and maternal skeletal muscle demands are met [18].

Fat is a major source of energy and aids in the absorption of fat-soluble vitamins and carotenoids. The developing brain of the fetus requires large amounts of docosahexaenoic acid (DHA), so adequate supplementation of essential fatty acids is recommended during pregnancy [18].

Vitamin A is important for gene expression and cell differentiation in the developing fetus [19].

Vitamin D maintains serum calcium and phosphorus concentrations and serves as a potent antiproliferative and prodifferentiation hormone [20].

Vitamin E is an antioxidant that prevents lipid peroxidation, especially for polyunsaturated fatty acids within the membrane phospholipids and plasma lipoproteins [21]. Blood concentrations increase during pregnancy and placental transfer appears constant.

Vitamin K is used as a coenzyme in protein synthesis for blood coagulation and bone metabolism. Data about its role during pregnancy is limited [19].

Thiamin is a coenzyme in metabolism of carbohydrates and branched-chain amino acids. The increased requirement during pregnancy is used for energy production both maternally and by the fetus [22].

Riboflavin is a coenzyme in oxidation–reduction reactions with additional needs during pregnancy to meet the growth and energy utilization by the fetus [22].

Niacin is required to form nicotinamide adenine dinucleotide and nicotinamide-adenine dinucleotide phosphate, plus biosynthesis of fatty acids and steroids [22].

Vitamin B_6 is involved in the metabolism of amino acids, glycogen, and sphingoid bases. B_6 coenzymes are needed for heme synthesis and transsulfuration breakdown of homocysteine to cysteine [22].

Folate functions in the metabolism of nucleic and amino acids, DNA synthesis, and cell division. Inadequate concentrations of folate can result in megablastic anemia [22].

Vitamin B_{12} is a coenzyme for the metabolism of fatty acids and in methyl transfer reactions. Absorption may decrease during pregnancy and vegan diets especially need supplementation of Vitamin B_{12} [22].

Pantothenic acid is a component of coenzyme A but little information is available about needs during pregnancy [22].

Biotin functions in carboxylation reactions with D-methylmalonyl-coenzyme A formation, which is dependent on adequate biotin [22].

Choline is a precursor to acetylcholine, phospholipids, and betaine. It is synthesized in the body but may be inadequate under certain conditions like pregnancy since large amounts are delivered to the fetus during pregnancy [22].

Sodium and chloride maintain the extracellular volume and serum osmolality, which do not usually require supplementation during pregnancy.

Potassium has influence on neural transmission, muscle contraction, and vascular tone. The adequate intake is the same for pregnant and nonpregnant women [23]. The high level of progesterone may help conserve potassium in pregnancy.

Calcium contributes to the strength of bones and teeth, along with mediating vascular contractions, vasodilation, muscle contraction, nerve transmission, and glandular secretions. Due to increased absorption efficiency in pregnancy, increased supplementation is not recommended unless bone degradation has occurred prior to pregnancy [20].

Phosphorus is essential in all tissues but due to enhanced absorption during pregnancy, no additional supplementation is recommended [20].

Magnesium is required in over 300 enzymes with the fetus demanding a significant amount. That demand usually requires additional supplementation [20].

Chromium improves insulin action but its need during pregnancy has not been accurately determined [19].

Copper is a component of metalloenzymes for reduction of oxygen. The fetus must accumulate copper during pregnancy and so intake of dietary and supplemental sources of copper need to be encouraged [19].

Fluoride can inhibit the initiation and progression of dental caries and stimulate new bone development. It crosses the placenta and gets incorporated into primary teeth. Supplementation during pregnancy is not supported [20].

Iodine is essential for thyroid hormones and regulates protein synthesis. Thyroid hormone is critical for myelination of the central nervous system and is very active during the prenatal period. Lack of iodine damages the developing brain and its deficiency leads to mental retardation, hypothyroidism, and goiter [19].

Iron is a component of proteins—heme, iron–sulfur, iron storage, and transport and iron-activated enzymes. Lack of iron during pregnancy can lead to perinatal mortality. Maternal anemia is also associated with premature delivery and low birth weight. The fetal need for iron is met at the expense of maternal stores so most women will need supplementation during pregnancy [19].

Manganese is needed for bone and amino acid metabolism. Data is very limited on its need in pregnancy [19].

Molybdenum is a cofactor in numerous enzymes like sulfite oxidase, xanthine oxidase, and aldehyde oxidase. No data is available about needs during pregnancy [19].

Selenium is important to regulate thyroid hormone action, defend against oxidative stress, and regulate redox status of vitamin C. The fetus stores selenoproteins during development so additional supplementation is recommended [19].

Zinc has regulatory function in over 100 enzymes. As the fetus develops, it stores zinc throughout the pregnancy and requirement increases substantially [19].

Major Foods and Nutrient Sources during Pregnancy

Sunlight: vitamin D—4,000 IU supplement daily

Eggs: protein, choline, lutein, and zeaxanthin

Salmon: protein, omega-3 fatty acids—eicosapentaenoic acid (EPA) and DHA

Dairy: protein, B vitamins, zinc (yogurt or kefir are better tolerated than whole milk)

Sweet potatoes: beta carotene, fiber

Greens: cooked spinach, asparagus for folate, fiber, vitamin K

Beef and chicken: protein, B vitamins, iron

Grass-fed beef liver: vitamin B_{12}, iron

Avocados: potassium, B vitamins, folate, monounsaturated fatty acids

Papaya: folate, beta carotene, vitamin C

CASE STUDY

TR is a 29-year-old female, 3 years postlapband, who has a 5-month-old male infant. During pregnancy: vomiting + food cravings. She had not eaten her favorite foods since lapband surgery, so she ate them and regained 60 lb.

Current weight: 253.8 lb., body mass index (BMI): 39.8, body fat: 49.5%.

24-hour food recall—breakfast: coffee "depends on mood" + sandwich or cake or cereal; lunch: subway sandwich; snack: crackers; dinner: steak or salad or beans, and rice.

With gastric banding she lived off of shakes and chili and did not eat pizza for 3 years!

Plan of Care: Nutrition counseling for lapband removal and preparation for gastric bypass. She is familiar with liquid diet but needs lifestyle change to prevent weight regain because she has found she loves pizza and sandwiches.

References

1. Milone M, De Placido G, Musella M, et al. Incidence of successful pregnancy after weight loss interventions in infertile women: A systematic review and meta-analysis of the literature. *Obes Surg* 2015 Dec 12;26(2):443–451.
2. Duval K, Langlois MF, Carranza-Mamane B, et al. The obesity-fertility protocol: A randomized controlled trial assessing clinical outcomes and costs of a transferable interdisciplinary lifestyle intervention, before and during pregnancy, in obese infertile women. *BMC Obesity* 2015;2:47.
3. Ciangura C, Nizard J, Poitou-Bernert C, et al. Pregnancy and bariatric surgery: Critical points. *J Gynecol Obstet Biol Reprod* 2015 Jun;44(6):496–502.
4. Shils ME, Olson JA, Shike M, et al. *Modern Nutrition in Health and Diseases*. Philadelphia, PA: Lippincott Williams & Wilkins, 2006, pp. 772–773.
5. Kakarla N, Dailey C, Marino T, et al. Pregnancy after gastric bypass surgery and internal hernia formation. *Am Coll Obstet Gyn* 2005 May;105:1195–1198.
6. Filip JE, Mattar SG, Bowers SP, et al. Internal hernia formation after laparoscopic Roux-en-Y gastric bypass for morbid obesity. *Am Surg* 2002;68:640–643.

7. Jacquemyn Y, Meesters J. Pregnancy as a risk factor for undertreatment after bariatric surgery. *BMJ Case Rep* 2014 Jan 9;bcr2013202779.
8. Chevrot A, Lesage N, Msika S, et al. Digestive surgical complications during pregnancy following bariatric surgery: Experience of a center for perinatology and obesity. *J Gynecol Obstet Biol Reprod* 2015 May 20;45(4):372–379.
9. Johansson K, Cnattingius S, Ingmar Näslund MD, et al. Outcomes of pregnancy after bariatric surgery. *N Engl J Med* 2015 Feb 26;372(9):814–824.
10. Pelizzo G, Calcaterra V, Fusillo M, et al. Malnutrition in pregnancy following bariatric surgery: Three clinical cases of fetal neural defects. *Nutr J* 2014 Jan 14;13:59.
11. Jans G, Matthys C, Bogaerts A, et al. Maternal micronutrient deficiencies and related adverse neonatal outcomes after bariatric surgery: A systematic review. *Adv Nutr* 2015 Jul 15;6(4):420–429.
12. Machado SN, Pereira S, Saboya C, et al. Influences of Roux-en-Y gastric bypass on the nutritional status of Vitamin A in pregnant woman: A comparative study. *Obes Surg* 2015 May 22;26(1):26–31.
13. Devlieger R, Guelinckx I, Jans G, et al. Micronutrient levels and supplement intake in pregnancy after bariatric surgery: A prospective cohort study. *PLOS One* 2014 Dec 3;9(12):e114192.
14. Chevrot A, Kayem G, Coupaye M, et al. Impact of bariatric surgery on fetal growth restriction: Experience of a perinatal and bariatric surgery center. *Am J Obstet Gynecol* 2015 Nov 25;214(5):655.e1–e7.
15. Dell' Agnolo CM, Cyr C, de Montigny, et al. Pregnancy after bariatric surgery: Obstetric and perinatal outcomes, and growth and development of children. *Obes Surg* 2015;25(11):2030–2039.
16. Manning S, Finer N, Elkalaawy M, et al. Timing of pregnancy in obese women after bariatric surgery. *Pregnancy Hypertens* 2014 July;4(3):235.
17. Andreasen LA, Nilas L, Kjaer MM. Operative complications during pregnancy after gastric bypass—A register-based cohort study. *Obes Surg* 2014;24:1634–1638.
18. Food and Nutrition Board, Institute of Medicine. *Dietary Reference Intakes for Energy, Carbohydrate, Fiber, Fat, Fatty Acids, Cholesterol, Protein, and Amino Acids.* Washington, DC: National Academy Press, 2002.
19. Food and Nutrition Board, Institute of Medicine. *Dietary Reference Intakes for Vitamin A, Vitamin K, Arsenic, Boron, Chromium, Copper, Iron, Manganese, Molybdenum, Nickel, Silicon, Vanadium, and Zinc.* Washington, DC: National Academy Press, 2001.
20. Food and Nutrition Board, Institute of Medicine. *Dietary Reference Intakes for Calcium, Phosphorus, Magnesium, Vitamin D, and Fluoride.* Washington, DC: National Academy Press, 1997.
21. Food and Nutrition Board, Institute of Medicine. *Dietary Reference Intake for Vitamin C, Vitamin E, Selenium and Carotenoids.* Washington, DC: National Academy Press, 2000.

22. Food and Nutrition Board, Institute of Medicine. *Dietary Reference Intake for Thiamin, Riboflavin, Niacin, Vitamin B6, Folate, Vitamin B12, Pantothenic Acid, Biotin and Choline*. Washington, DC: National Academy Press, 1998.

23. Food and Nutrition Board, Institute of Medicine. *Dietary Reference Intakes for Water, Potassium, Sodium, Chloride and Sulfate*. Washington, DC: National Academy Press, 2004.

10
Digestive Health

Eat less—exercise more is the mantra for managing the obesity crisis, yet common sense should awaken health-care professionals to the fact that an 1,800 cal standard American diet of low-fat proteins, vegetables, fruits, and whole grains will produce far different weight management than an 1,800 cal diet of Oreos, potato chips, and soda.

A study in the *American Journal of Clinical Nutrition* in 2013 indicated that Americans were eating fewer calories between 2003 and 2010 but obesity rates have not reduced [1]. The calories in/calories out equation is not relevant to answer the challenge of obesity that is taking over the world.

The human body is a complex network of trillions of microorganisms that live on us and in us. This garden of life that Gerald E. Mullin, MD, describes in *The Gut Balance Revolution* is composed of viruses, bacteria, and fungi called the microbiome [2]. These microbes are responsible for breaking down fruits and vegetables, vitamin, and mineral absorption, and production of short-chain fatty acids to protect gut immunity and defend against foreign invaders while supporting detoxification and modulating mood and nervous system responses.

Food Digestion

The human gastrointestinal (GI) tract is a complex system that ranges from the mouth to the anus and transforms ingested food into nutrients that can be absorbed by the body to maintain the health of each individual. But variations between individuals may lead to large differences in responses during the digestive process based on the enzymatic and pH conditions found in the mouth, stomach, and intestine [3].

In the mouth, the mastication and shearing action of the tongue causes degradation of the ingested bite of food. Saliva lubricates and the mixing action of the tongue and palate transforms the food into a bolus for swallowing. Saliva is about 99% water with various electrolytes—sodium, potassium, calcium, and bicarbonate—mucins, enzymes, and amylase to begin the breakdown of starch. The bolus is swallowed and passes through the esophagus where it moves via peristaltic contractions until it enters the stomach.

The stomach storage area is where the bolus is mixed with gastric secretions, enzymes (pepsin, gastric lipase), intrinsic factor, and hydrochloric acid at a pH of 1.5–2.0. At the distal end of the stomach, the pylorus acts as a valve to allow particles to enter the small intestine.

In the small intestine, the digested food (now called chyme) is mixed with intestinal secretions to gradually increase the alkalinity and allow pancreatic enzymes (lipase, amylase, amyloglucosidase, trypsin, phospholipase A, chymotrypsin, carboxypeptidase, and elastase) to act while bile salts digest lipids [4,5].

Nutrients in the small intestine diffuse through the mucus layer over the gut wall and are transported from the lumen through the cell membrane to the enterocytes and eventually to the blood [4,6].

The large intestine is the body's fermenter and absorption of water and some vitamins occurs here while waste material is converted into feces. Fermentation of unabsorbed food particles occurs by a large microbial population.

Microbiome of the Gut

Millions of microbes enter the body at every meal and the digestive tract is a warm space filled with lots of compounds for microbes to grow on. The microbiome in each individual gets established at birth during delivery with the bacteria found in the vagina. Cesarean section delivery does not provide the same microbiome advantages.

Changes in the diet can also produce modifications in the gut microbiome. Numerous studies have questioned the use of high-protein diets due to reduced butyrate producing bacteria and increased cadaverine, spermine, and sulfide in the feces [7–9]. Mu et al. discuss how different dietary food choices can produce changes to the microbial community caused by a high-protein diet that alters the microbial metabolites in the colons of rats compared with a normal protein diet [10].

Body weight can be influenced by the microbiome in the gut according to a twin study by researchers at King's College London and Cornell University [11]. The National Institute of Health (NIH)-funded study accessed the genetics of microbes in over 1,000 fecal samples from 416 pairs of twins. Specific types of microbes were found to be more similar in identical twins than nonidentical twins. Health-promoting bacteria were more abundant in those with a low-body weight, which suggested to the researchers that microbes may help prevent or reduce obesity.

Sex-dependent differences in microbes living in the gut were studied at the University of Texas, Austin. Investigators found that fish and mice data showed microbe differences between males and females despite identical diets [12]. They concluded that the difference between them was related to the hormonal influence on gut microbes or the difference in the immune function that affected which microbes lived or died. Dr. Daniel Bolnick, professor in the University's College of Natural Sciences, stated, "This means that most of the research that's being done on lab mice—we need to treat with kid gloves."

Microbiome Health

Food choices influence the body in far greater ways than just energy in/energy out. The GI tract from the mouth to anus consists of over 1,000 different species of microbes that live and flourish as the largest and most diverse microbiome in the human body. Research on this topic is still in its infancy and some call the GI tract the hidden brain or second brain.

Research has shown that the microbiome plays an important role in various diseases like irritable bowel syndrome (IBS), inflammatory bowel disease (IBD or Crohn's disease, ulcerative colitis), colorectal cancer, diabetes, allergic reactions, and obesity in addition to mood and behavior disorders. The gut microbiome evolves within the individual over time and is dependent on dietary habits, lifestyle, environmental factors, stress, and age [13].

Dysbiosis or disruption of the healthy microbiota is considered the trigger for many diseases. Studies have shown that the American diet—high-fat, low-plant foods, high-animal fat—produces a less diverse GI microbiome [14]. A high-fiber diet with a variety of plant foods promotes variety and increases diversity in microbiota.

Different people have different microbiota combinations that can have a dramatic impact on their weight and health. The consensus of numerous studies is that weight gain is caused by an abundance of Firmicute bacteria while leanness is associated with *Bacteroides* bacteria [15]. Follow-up research has focused on why firmicutes are associated with obesity. It appears that they impact carbohydrate and fat metabolism [16].

Studies have shown that firmicute levels reduce in obese individuals who undergo gastric bypass surgery [17]. The improvement in gut microbiota balance appears soon after gastric bypass surgery and seems to contribute to insulin sensitivity before any substantial weight is lost.

Obesity and GI Disorders

The World Health Organization (WHO) estimated that 1.5 billion adults were overweight in 2008 with a body mass index (BMI) of 25 kg/m^2 or higher [18]. The Centers for Disease Control and Prevention in 2013 ranked the U.S. population in 2009–2010 as 69.2% overweight and 35.9% obese [19]. GI disorders have a high prevalence in this population [20].

Gut inflammation caused by cytokines can influence mood and cognition as well as alterations in the stomach and intestines presenting as IBS, gastroesophageal reflux disease (GERD), ulcers, or Crohn's disease, which can be secondary disorders to obesity. These inflammatory diseases can be caused from food intolerances and/or inadequate microbiota balance.

Many bariatric candidates present with bloating and abdominal pain after eating. Common triggers to digestive inflammation are grain and dairy foods. Since the gut contains an estimated 70%–80% of the immune system, this represents the largest contact area that the human body has with the external world. The lymphoid tissue surrounding the intestines—the gut associated lymphoid tissue (GALT)—forms the largest immune organ in the body.

A continuous intake of reactive substances causes inflammation in the intestinal tissue, which spreads to other tissues affecting the hormonal and nervous system [21]. Food intolerances can be caused by

poor diet habits, stress, and fatigue and can be associated with elevated inflammation markers like C-reactive protein (CRP). Lactose,
gluten, and fructose intolerances can be due to an enzyme deficiency
while celiac disease is a genetic factor [22].

Helicobacter Pylori

Helicobacter pylori (*H. pylori*) is a bacteria that lives in the digestive
tract and can cause ulcers in the stomach or upper small intestine.
The bacterial inflammation can lead to inflammation and infections
that prevent food from moving through the digestive tract. Treatment
prior to surgery can help relieve the gut bloating and stomach pains.

Low-Inflammation Diet

A low-inflammation diet may be needed by bariatric surgery candidates to reduce dysbiosis and cytokine activity pre- and postsurgery.
An example of a low-inflammation meal plan follows:

Breakfast	Ground pork sausage or pork chop
	Papaya and banana fruit cup
	Herbal tea or black coffee
Lunch	Poached salmon or cod
	Boiled potato and avocado or Basmati rice and olive oil
	Vegetable soup or salad
	Herbal tea or green tea
Dinner	Baked chicken or turkey
	Baked sweet potato with olive oil
	Asparagus or green beans
	Poached pear
	Water
Snacks	Mashed fresh avocado with carrot and celery sticks

Foods to exclude: chocolate, ketchup, soy sauce, barbecue (BBQ)
sauce, peanuts, tree nuts, cold cuts, frankfurters, shellfish, dairy foods,
eggs, wheat, corn, barley, spelt, kamut, oats.

- Raw fruit (except banana) are not recommended in gut healing. Frozen fruits are a better choice until raw can be tolerated.

- Salad greens, tomatoes, onions, garlic consumed in small amounts are usually tolerated. Minimum amounts of broccoli, Brussels sprouts, kale need to be added slowly to access tolerance.

4-R Program

The goal in successful weight management postsurgery needs to include a 4-R approach to establishing and maintaining a healthy gut: Remove, Replace, Reinoculate, and Repair.

- Remove from the diet any foods that interfere with a healthy microbiota balance that could cause bad microbiota growth—sugar, *trans* fats, soy, gluten, dairy (if lactose intolerant or sensitive).
- Replace with foods from low-inflammation diet—vegetables, fruits, lean proteins, healthy fats like avocado and olive oil.
- Reinoculate with probiotics and digestive enzymes.
- Repair the microbiota with adequate dietary supplements and amino acids.

Bariatric surgery candidates can be introduced to the 4-R program in support groups in preparation for surgery. Many of them could profit from this approach to changing their diet for a better outcome instead of thinking the surgery will be all that they will need to lose weight.

Carswell and Vincent followed Roux-en-Y Gastric Bypass (RYGB) patients and found few abnormalities in malabsorption of fats and sugars indicating diet modification to be critical for success in bariatric surgery [23].

Sugar and Artificial Sweeteners

When the gut microbiome becomes imbalanced, weight gain can result from inflammation leading to insulin resistance, visceral adipose tissue deposits (belly fat), and leptin resistance. Sugar is a major food source that causes inflammation or gut dysbiosis. The average American eats about 150 lb. of sugar annually from beet, corn, and cane sweeteners. The WHO now recommends that no more than 5% of the daily calories should come from added sugars [24]. The Centers for Disease Control and Prevention indicate that Americans currently consume an average of 15%–20% of their daily calories from added sugar [24].

High-sugar intake has been linked to type 2 diabetes, obesity, fatty liver disease, stroke, and cardiovascular disorders [25]. A study at the University of Southern California has shown that adolescent rats that freely consumed large quantities of sugar liquids experienced memory problems and brain inflammation along with prediabetes symptoms [26]. They concluded that a diet high in added sugars not only can lead to weight gain and metabolic disturbances but can also impact neural function and cognitive ability.

Noncalorie artificial sweeteners are some of the most widely used food additives worldwide. Scientific data is sparse on their safety but one study demonstrated that their consumption drove development of glucose intolerance through an alteration in the gut microbiota [27].

Fats

Trans fatty acids play a role in the inflammatory process by stimulating the release of cytokines. They are produced industrially through partial hydrogenation of liquid plant oils and are directly related to all-cause mortality in the *British Medical Journal* [28]. A Danish study identified a dietary intake of 5 g of *trans* fat as causing a 25% increased risk of ischemic heart disease due to inflammatory cytokines [29]. A serving of French fries and chicken nuggets from McDonald's was evaluated from several countries showing a possible consumption of 10–25 g *trans* fatty acids in one day.

According to data published in the *British Journal of Nutrition*, *trans* fats 18:2 fatty acids were integrated into human aortic endothelial at twice the rate as *cis* 18:2 fatty acids, which caused cells to clump together and bind to the arterial walls. This response stimulates the release of proinflammatory cytokines throughout the body.

Probiotics

Probiotics can offer healthy balance to GI microbiota by supplying protection against pathogenic bacteria, facilitating nutrient absorption, and harmonizing microorganisms disrupted by stress, disease, poor nutrition, and medications. The microbiota within the gut consists of native indigenous species but a highly processed food diet can result in reduced variety and balance.

Bacteria like *lactobacilli* and *bifidobacteria* help the body resist bad bacteria while aiding digestion and nutrient absorption. Probiotics also help to strengthen the barrier function of the intestinal wall in addition to improving immunity by stimulating natural killer and T cells.

According to Liska et al. [30] the common bacteria species found in the GI tract are listed as follows:

Stomach	*Lactobacilli*
Small Intestine	*Lactobacilli*
	Streptococci
	Enterobacteria
	Bacteroides
Large Intestine	*Bacteroides*
	Fusobacterium
	Enterococcus faecalis
	Lactobacilli
	Staphylococcus aureus
	Clostridium
	Enterobacteria
	Klebsiella
	Eubacteria
	Bifidobacteria
	Streptococci
	Pseudomonas
	Salmonella
Feces	*Bacteroides*
	Bifidobacteria
	Eubacteria
	Coliforms
	E. faecalis

Bacterial imbalance in the gut can affect other organ systems and can result in joint inflammation to osteoporosis and cancer. To restore balance, probiotic supplementation is helpful. In the early 1900s,

Nobel laureate Eli Metchnikoff reported favorable health effects from fermented milk products. In 1965, Lilly and Stillwell introduced the term "probiotics" for growth promoting factors produced by microorganisms. Fuller in 1989 described probiotics as live microbial feed supplements which benefited intestinal balance. The International Life Sciences Institute in 2001 defined probiotics as, "viable microbial food supplements which beneficially influence the health of humans" [31].

Probiotics consist of lactic acid producing species, nonlactic acid producing bacterial species, and nonpathogenic yeast. To achieve the best results from adding probiotics to the dietary supplement regime, select a full spectrum probiotic that resides in the small and large intestine. Some commercial products are made nondairy, heat stable, and stomach acid-resistant so they offer the full benefit.

A list of several probiotic species commonly used in dietary supplements follows [32].

- *Lactobacillus* is a beneficial organism and is the most prominent microorganism found in the small intestine. It is known to implant itself on the intestinal wall, and is also found in the lining of the vagina, cervix, and urethra. It performs many critical functions including inhibiting pathogenic organisms and preventing them from multiplying and colonizing. More than 100 species are identified. The commonly used species in probiotics are as follows:

    Lactobacillus acidophilus
    Lactobacillus brevis
    Lactobacillus bulgaricus
    Lactobacillus casei
    Lactobacillus crispatus
    Lactobacillus fermentum
    Lactobacillus gasseri
    Lactobacillus helveticus
    Lactobacillus jensenii
    Lactobacillus johnsonii
    Lactobacillus paracasei
    Lactobacillus plantarum
    Lactobacillus rhamnoses
    Lactobacillus salivarius

- *Bifidobacterium* is a prominent probiotic microorganism that takes up residence primarily in the mucous membrane lining of the large intestines and the vaginal tract. *Bifidobacterium bifidum* is important in preventing colonization of invading pathogenic bacteria by attaching to the intestinal wall and crowding out unfriendly bacteria and yeast. *Bifidobacteria* enhance the assimilation and metabolism of minerals—iron, calcium, and magnesium. Bifidobacteria is a genus of lactic acid producing bacteria that is anaerobic and found predominately in the large intestine. The most common species are the following:

    Bifidobacterium adolescentis
    Bifidobacterium animalis
    Bifidobacterium bifidum
    Bifidobacterium breve
    Bifidobacterium infantis
    Bifidobacterium lactis
    Bifidobacterium longum
    Bifidobacterium thermophilum

- *Streptococcus* species are not usually pathogenic but one anaerobic species *Streptococcus thermophilus* is known to promote health and is found in yogurt cultures with *L. bulgaricus*. *L. bulgaricus* is considered a transient microorganism that does not implant in the intestinal tract but provides important protective and supplemental roles. This is the organism used to ferment natural yogurt.

- *Bacillus* species are nonlactic acid producing probiotics that are commonly found in soil and water. Spores of bacillus are used as probiotics but controversy surrounds their use according to Dr. Steven Olmstead [32].

- Yeast probiotics or *Saccharomyces* is a genus of 7–10 species with only *Saccharomyces boulardi* being used as a probiotic. It is unaffected by gastric acid and bile so it can proliferate throughout the GI tract for diarrhea and *Clostridium difficile*-associated disorders. It has been shown to inhibit *candida* adhesion and reduce colonization.

Key Functions of Specific Probiotic Species

- *L. bulgaricus* is considered a transient microorganism that does not implant in the intestinal tract but provides important protective and supplemental roles. This is the organism used to ferment natural yogurt.
- *L. plantarum* plays a role in the secretion of naturally occurring antibiotic lactolin. It is also known to have the ability to synthesize L-lysine for beneficial antiviral activity.
- *B. infantis* is the primary organism in the intestines of infants and also in the vaginal tract.

As Rob Knight in his TED book *Follow Your Gut—The enormous impact of tiny microbes* states: "The biggest problem is that many people seemed to assume that any probiotic will do. We wouldn't do this for anything else" [33]. Selecting a probiotic with a randomized, controlled trial recommendation is slim to none because few exist. Many people choose "live yogurt" but as clinical data shows, many yogurts have limited to no live cultures by the time they get consumed [34,35].

References

1. Ford ES, Dietz WH. Trends in energy intake among adults in the United States: Findings from NHANES. *Amer J Clin Nutr* 2013;97:848–853.
2. Mullin GE. *The Gut Balance Revolution*. Emmaus, PA: Rodale, 2015, p. 7.
3. Bornhorst GM, Gouseti O, Wickham MS, et al. Engineering digestion: Multiscale process of food digestion. *J Food Sci* 2016; 81(3):R534–R543.
4. Barrett KE. *Gastrointestinal Physiology*, Second Edition. New York, NY: McGraw Hill Medical, 2013.
5. Bornhorst GM, Singh RP. Gastric digestion in vivo and in vitro: How the structural aspects of food influence the digestive process. *Ann Rev Food Sci Tech* 2014;5:111–132.
6. Guyton AC, Hall JE. *Textbook of Medical Physiology*. Philadelphia, PA: Elsevier-Sanders, 2006.
7. Louis P, Hold GL, Flint HJ. The gut microbiota, bacterial metabolites and colorectal cancer. *Nat Rev Microbiol* 2014;12:661–672.
8. Russell WR, Gratz SW, Duncan SH, et al. High protein, reduced carbohydrate weight loss diets promote metabolic profiles likely to be detrimental to colonic health. *Am J Clin Nutr* 2011;93:1062–1072.
9. Duncan SH, Belenguer A, Holtrop G, et al. Reduced dietary intake of carbohydrates by obese subjects results in decreased concentrations of butyrate and butyrate-producing bacteria in feces. *Appl Environ Microbiol* 2007;73:1073–1078.

10. Mu C, Yang Y, Luo Z, et al. The colonic microbiome and epithelial transciption are altered in rats fed a high protein diet compared with a normal protein diet. *J Nutr* 2016;3(146):474–483.

11. King's College London. Body weight heavily influenced by gut microbes: Genes shape body weight by affecting gut microbes. *ScienceDaily*. Available at: www.sciencedaily.com/releases/2014/11/141106132204.htm.

12. Bolnick D I, Snowberg LK, Hirsch PE, et al. Individual diet has sex-dependent effects on vertebrate gut microbiota. Nat Commun 2014 July 29;5:4500.

13. Guinane CM, Cotter PD. Role of gut microbiota and chronic gastro-intestinal disease: Understanding a hidden metabolic organ. *Therap Adv Gastroenterol* 2013;6(4):2295–2308.

14. Graf D, Di Cagno R, Fak F, et al. Contribution of diet to the composition of the human gut microbiota. *Microb Ecol Hum Dis* 2015;26:1651–2235.

15. Ley RE, Turnbaugh PJ, Klein S, et al. Microbial ecology: Human gut microbes associated with obesity. *Nature* 2006;444:1022–1023.

16. Turnbaugh PJ, Hamady M, Yatsunenko T, et al. A core gut microbiome in obese and lean twins. *Nature* 2009;457:480–484.

17. Patel RT, Shukla AP, Ahn SM, et al. Surgical control of obesity and diabetes: The role on intestinal vs gastric mechanisms in the regulation of body weight and glucose homeostasis. *Obesity* 2014;22(1):159–169.

18. World Health Organization. *Obesity and Overweight*. Geneva, Switzerland: World Health Organization 2013. Available at: http://www.who-int/mediacentre/factsheets.

19. Centers for Disease Control and Prevention. 2013. Available at: http://www.cdc.gov/obesity/adult/index.

20. Bouchoucha M, Fysekidis M, Julia C, et al. Functional gastrointestinal disorders in obese patients—The importance of the enrollment source. *Obes Surg* 2015;25:2143–2552.

21. Wan-Wan L, Karin M. A cytokine-related link between innate immunity, inflammation and cancer. *J Clin Invest* 2007;117(5):1175–1183.

22. Tlaskalova-Hogenova T, Tucková L, Stepánková R, et al. Involvement of innate immunity in the development of inflammatory and autoimmune diseases. *Ann NY Acad Sci* 2005;1051:787–798.

23. Carswell KA, Vincent RP, Belgaumkar AP, et al. The effect of bariatric surgery on intestinal absorption and transit time. *Obes Surg* 2014;24:796–805.

24. Schmidt LA. New unsweetened truths about sugar. *JAMA Internal Med* 2014;17:525–526.

25. Turnbaugh PJ, Ridaura VK, Faith JJ, et al. The effects of diet on the human gut microbiome: A metagenomic analysis in humanized gnotobiotic mice. *Sci Trans Med* 2009;1:6.

26. Hsu TM, Konanur VR, Taing L, et al. Effects of sucrose and high fructose corn syrup consumption on spatial memory function and hippocaampal neurinflammation in adolescent rats. *Hippocampus* 2014 Sept 20;25(2):227–239.

27. Suez J, Korem T, Zeevi D, et al. Artificial sweeteners induce glucose intolerance by altering the gut microbiota. *Nature* 2014 Oct 9;514(7521):181–186.

28. deSouza RJ, Mente A, Maroleanu A, et al. Intake of saturated and trans unsaturated fatty acids and risk of all cause mortality, cardiovascular disease, Type 2 diabetes: Systemic review and meta-analysis of observational studies. *BMJ* 2015 Aug 12;351:h3978.

29. Stender S, Dyerberg J. High levels of industrial produced trans fat in popular fast food. *NEJ Med* 2006;354:1650–1652.

30. Liska D, Quinn S, Lukaczer, et al. Clinical Nutrition—A Functional Approach. Washington, DC: Institute for Functional Medicine, 2004, p. 206.

31. Olmstead S, Snodgrass R, Meiss D, et al. *Making Sense of Probiotics.* Reno, NV: Klaire Labs Technical Summary.

32. Olmstead SF. *Newsletter.* Reno, NV: Prothera, Inc., 2013.

33. Knight B. *Follow Your Gut—The Enormous Impact of Tiny Microbes. TED Books.* New York, NY: Simon and Schuster, 2015.

34. Merenstein DJ, Foster J, D'Amico F. A randomized clinical trial measuring the influence of kefir on antibiotic-associated diarrhea: Measuring the influence of kefir (milk) study. *Arch Pediatr Adolesc Med* 2009 Aug 8;163:750–754.

35. Beniwal RS. A randomized trial of yogurt for prevention of antibiotic-associated diarrhea. *Dig Dis Sci* 2003 Oct;48(10):2077–2082.

11
DETOXIFICATION

We live in a toxic world and as Alan Gaby, MD, in *Nutritional Medicine* states "In modern times, humans, are exposed to tens of thousands of harmful or potentially harmful compounds, including pesticides, herbicides, solvents, petrochemicals, heavy metals and plastics" [1]. Most of these substances are fat soluble and are found throughout the body in the adipose tissue. The Environmental Protection Agency in 1982 reported that 20 toxic compounds were found in 76%–100% of the adipose tissue samples taken from cadavers and elective surgery patients from throughout the United States [1].

Reduction of adipose tissue releases these compounds into the systemic circulation, which can be detrimental to neurological function. Continued exposure to toxin release throughout bariatric surgery weight loss could play a role in the pathogenesis of autoimmune disorders like systemic lupus erythematosus, dementia, Alzheimer's, and Parkinson's disease. Reduction of the toxic load can also lead to chronic fatigue, thyroiditis, rheumatoid arthritis, other connective tissue disorders, and multiple sclerosis [1–3].

A number of commercial laboratories offer testing for toxic body burden levels of pesticides, polychlorinated biphenyls (PCBs), solvents, heavy metals, and other toxins [4]. Environmental medicine denotes that toxic chemicals contribute to chronic illness and a detoxification regime can enhance well-being by stabilizing or reversing disease through a program of exercise and low-grade hyperthermia (sauna) to stimulate the release of toxic chemicals from storage in fat tissue [5]. Some chemicals are removed through sweat and others are transported to the liver for conversion to water-soluble compounds that exit the body in the feces and urine. Further information is available at the Walter Crinnion, ND, website [6].

The study of detoxification processes in the body and influences on health is a young field of science but research is helping clinicians understand the complexities of cytochrome P_{450} in Phase 1 and conjugation during Phase 2. In the 1970s cytochrome P_{450} was found in the liver and researchers discovered it was responsible for converting lipophilic (fat stored) toxins into intermediates that were water-soluble. As research continued into the 1980s and 1990s, investigators uncovered the enzymes in the liver, called conjugases, that allowed drugs and xenobiotics to be excreted from the body [7].

Lab Assessments of Detoxification

Some measures of metabolic effects found on the comprehensive metabolic panel (CMP) can show impaired detoxification function [8].

- UREA (blood urea nitrogen or BUN) is a detoxified form of ammonia. A high value may indicate ammonia loading exceeding urea production capacity
- AMMONIA markers may indicate urea cycle capacity is exceeded or high values signal liver dysfunction
- BILIRUBIN elevation is caused by impaired glucuronidation and drug monitoring is needed (i.e., acetaminophen)
- CREATININE increase can lead to kidney damage due to autoimmune diseases, congestive heart failure, atherosclerosis, or diabetes complications

Nutrition Influence in Detoxification

Dr. Paul Talalay at Johns Hopkins University School of Medicine revealed how select phytochemicals in plant foods can modify Phase 1 and Phase 2 enzyme systems [7]. Chemicals in foods like green tea, onions, garlic, chlorophyll, broccoli, and other cruciferous vegetables act to improve detoxification [9]. Meal plans that use liberal amounts of these foods presurgery can aid the detoxification process.

Therapies to improve detoxification traditionally have been in a clinical setting so that a regulated diet, fasting, and sauna therapy could be closely supervised but this is not cost effective in many clinics so a home-based program can be designed for bariatric surgery candidates who could benefit from

- Improved gut functioning
- Heavy metal reduction (mercury, aluminum, cadmium, arsenic, lead)
- Decreased atrazine, bisphenol A, toluene, PCBs, and organo-phosphates stored in fat cells

Toxic metal and gastrointestinal function testing can be done to evaluate need and efficacy [4].

Fasting

A 1- or 2-day water fast can be a safe and effective way to regenerate weight loss efforts. Calorie restriction and fasting help to reduce hypertension, diabetes, and joint pain [10–12]. High glucose and insulin damage the mitochondria and calorie restriction reduces the oxidative stress in the mitochondria [13]. Fasting for a short period of time also improves liver function for lipid metabolism and nonalcoholic steatohepatitis (NASH). Cognition and immune function also benefit from calorie restriction [14,15].

Nutrition during Detoxification

After a 1- to 2-day fast, a low-inflammation diet of rice, frozen fruit, and steamed vegetables is followed for 4–5 days to reduce digestive problems and joint pain [16]. Raw vegetables, fresh fruit, and a variety of protein foods can be added after the first week. Food choices need to be based on whole foods—lots of vegetables, fruits, and fiber to increase detoxification. Olive oil and lean, unprocessed meat/poultry/fish, and eggs should be eaten daily. Undenatured whey protein or free amino acids support glutathione synthesis and add variety to protein choices at breakfast and snacks.

Exercise and Rest

Exercise increases the lymphatic flow and induces sweating for improved metabolism and detoxification efficiency. Proper sleep and relaxation is important during any detoxification program—whether it is a 1-day fast per week or a 5-day fast and detoxification regime.

Sauna or Hydrotherapy

Sauna therapy supports the removal of fat-soluble toxins but needs to be tailored to the individual. Medical studies on the effectiveness of sauna and hydrotherapy have not been done but it stimulates symptom relief by mechanisms not fully being understood [17].

Heat shock proteins (HSPs) are used by cells to counteract potentially harmful oxidizing proteins that interfere with cell repair. HSPs are induced by heat from the sauna by increasing core temperature for short periods. As the body adapts to these HSPs, plasma volume, and blood flow to the heart and muscles increase along with stimulation of human growth hormone [18].

Saunas are a warming and relaxing therapeutic way to experience detoxification for toxins, body fat reduction, and boosting metabolism.

- 15 minutes of infrared sauna have been shown to improve capillary function, revitalize circulatory systems, and increase cell metabolism.
- Infrared energy improves immune function and enhances cell regeneration.
- The human body is 60%–70% water and sauna heat causes the body's water molecules to dilate capillaries and increase pH within the body to reduce acidity and remove toxins [19].

Sauna temperatures should not exceed 150°F–180°F for 15–20 minutes one or two times per day during a detoxification program. No alcohol is allowed and 8 oz. of water pre- and post-sauna is recommended with a rest or laying down period of 5–10 minutes after each session. The cool down after a sauna can be achieved by towel drying and/or warm shower. Cooling down with a cold shower or water plunge has been called a "healthy stress" because it may increase glutathione and lower uric acid but caution is advised for those with hypertension and obesity [20,21].

Women who are pregnant are advised to use caution when using a sauna. Individuals with a history of elevated blood pressure, heat exhaustion, stroke, aortic stenosis, or fainting should also use caution when considering the use of sauna therapy.

Sauna therapy is recommended to be continued weekly for at least a month as the detoxification process continues to improve the gastro-intestinal tract, liver function, and immune system [18].

Implications for Bariatric Surgery Patients

Bariatric surgery candidates are anxious to lose as much weight as possible as a result of the surgery. Few of them realize the implications of the toxic burden caused from adipose tissue reduction. Modern lifestyles and lack of laboratory testing have not provided insight into the importance of detoxification, but organ systems beyond the imbalanced intestinal flora can all function more efficiently from a toxic clean-up. The awareness and functioning of interconnectiveness of the gut, brain, liver, and immune systems can provide better weight loss potential for all bariatric surgery patients.

References

1. Gaby AR. *Nutritional Medicine*. Concord, NH: Fritz Perlberg Publishing, 2011, pp. 1292–1294.
2. Steventon GB, Heafield MT, Waring RH, et al. Xenobiotic metabolism in Parkinson's disease. *Neurology* 1989;39:883–887.
3. Steventon GB, Heafield MT, Sturman S, et al. Xenobiotic metabolism in Alzheimer's disease. *Neurology* 1990;40:1095–1098.
4. Laboratories offering testing. Doctor's Data, Inc. Available at: www.doctorsdata.com; Genova Diagnostics Inc. Available at: www.gdx.net.
5. Crinnion WJ. Results of a decade of naturopathic treatment for environmental illnesses: A review of clinical records. *J Naturopathic Med* 1997;7:21–27.
6. Crinnion W. website. Available at: www.crinnionmedical.com.
7. Lyon M, Bland J, Jones DS. Clinical approaches to detoxification and biotransformation. In: Jones DS, ed. *Textbook of Functional Medicine*. Gig Harbor, WA: Institute of functional medicine, 2005, pp. 543–578.
8. Lord RS, Bralley JA, eds. *Laboratory Evaluations for Integrative and Functional Medicine*, Second Edition. Duluth, GA: Metametrix Institute, 2008, pp. 490–501.
9. Shapiro TA, Fahey JW, Wade KL, et al. Chemoprotective glucosinolates and isothiocyanates of broccoli sprouts: Metabolism and excretion in humans. *Cancer Epidemiol Biomarkers Prev* 2001;10:501–508.
10. Michalsen A, Weidenhammer W, Melchart D, et al. Short-term therapeutic fasting in the treatment of chronic pain and fatigue

syndromes—Well-being and side effects with and without mineral supplements. *Forsch Komplementarmed Klass Naturheilkd* 2002;9:221–227. [Translated from German]

11. McCarthy MF. A preliminary fast may potentiate response to a subsequent low-salt, low fat-vegan diet in the management of hypertension—Fasting as a strategy for breaking metabolic vicious cycles. *Med Hypotheses* 2003;60:624–633.

12. Iwashige K, Kouda K, Kouda M, et al. Calorie restricted diet and urinary pentosidine in patients with rheumatoid arthritis. *J Physiol Anthropol Appl Human Sci* 2004;23:19–24.

13. Merry BJ. Oxidative stress and mitochondrial function with aging—The effects of calorie restriction. *Aging Cell* 2004;3:7–12.

14. Mules MF, Demuro, Mulas C, G et al. Dietary restriction counteracts age-related changes in cholesterol metabolism in the rat. *Mech Ageing Dev* 2005;126:648–654.

15. Bray T, Taylor C. Tissue glutathione, nutrition, and oxidative stress. *Can J Physiol Pharmacol* 1993;71:746–751.

16. Adam O. Anti-inflammatory diet and rheumatic diseases. *Eur J Clin Nutr* 1995;49:703–717.

17. Jones DS ed. *Textbook of Functional Medicine.* Gig Harbor, WA: Institute of Functional Medicine, 2005, pp. 161–162.

18. Selsby JT, Rother S, Tsuda SJ, et al. Intermittent hyperthermia enhances skeletal muscle regrowth and attenuates oxidative damage following reloading. *J Appl Physiol (1985)* 2007 Apr;102(4):1702–1707.

19. Scoon GS, Hopkins WG, Mayhew S, et al. Effect of post-exercise sauna bathing on the endurance performance of competitive male runners. *J Sci Med Sport* 2007 Aug; 10(4):259–262.

20. Kukkonen-Harjula K, Oja P, Laustiola K, Vuori I, et al. Haemodynamic and hormonal responses to heat exposure in a Finnish sauna bath. *Eur J Appl Physiol Occup Physiol* 1989;58(5):543–550.

21. Fortney L. Sauna-induced sweating offers many health benefits. *U Wis Sch Med & Pub Health News feed* Jan 3, 2011.

12
LIFESTYLE CHANGES

As Thomas A. Farley, in a *New York Times Op-Ed*, stated, "There is good news in the fight against obesity: Rates are finally falling in young children. The bad news? They're continuing to rise to new heights in adults" [1].

Bariatric surgery offers each patient a **beginning**, but they need to change their values, habits, and set realistic goals to insure success. Motivational interviewing by the health-care team can help bring about changes and goal setting [2].

All habits have three things in common: (1) A cue or trigger, (2) a routine/reaction behavior, and (3) the reward. Repetition of this habit brings a feel good response from dopamine, which encourages repeat behavior. Choosing a new behavior is like taking a different road than the well-known paved road a person has always taken.

Bariatric patients know they need to change unhealthy behaviors but many lack the skills to set realistic goals and prepare for new behaviors. Eating habits, exercise, sleep, stress management, and mood issues can seem overwhelming unless family and group support can offer solace. Educators can provide the **SMART** goal setting format for bariatric weight loss patients to help them feel empowered and personalize their plan.

- **S** = specific eating and exercise goals (e.g., I will limit my snacking to only approved choices and will walk 30 minutes after dinner three times weekly)
- **M** = measure success by pounds lost and minutes per week of exercise completed (e.g., I will lose 2 lb. per week and increase exercise to four times per week if that weight loss is not achieved)
- **A** = achievable sleep pattern to enhance weight loss and immune function (e.g., I will be in bed by 10 PM for 8 hours of sleep each night)

- **R** = relaxation to overcome stress in daily life (e.g., I will join yoga class and practice daily)
- **T** = time for fun and personal reflection on success (e.g., when I have lost 25 lb., a trip to Disney World will be planned)

Eating Mindfully

The ancient Buddhist practice of mindfulness is the state of being present in the moment while noticing and accepting all that surrounds you in a nonjudgmental manner. Bariatric surgery patients need to learn to not go through a meal or snack on autopilot but paying attention to every bite they consume. Mindful eating means

- Think about your food choices.
- Examine why you are eating.
- Taste your food with all your senses.
- Eat slowly so that a feeling of satiety can be felt.

Distractions can occur when schedules get too busy or grocery shopping has been skipped or the refrigerator is bare. Mindful eating is more achievable when the pantry and refrigerator are organized, healthy food choices are available, and the food environment is conducive to new habits such as the following:

- Smaller plates and bowls are used for reduced portions.
- Food is put away and out of sight (except for ripening fruit and avocados)
- Healthy food is at eye level in the cabinet or refrigerator.
- Distractions are eliminated when eating. They result in eating more and faster—television, computer, cell phone.
- "Junk food" and "trigger foods" are kept out of the home.
- Use a grocery list and plan ahead.
- Keep a food journal or log to access how much processed food or restaurant eating goes on.

An example of a mindful eating log that can be used to help lead to better eating habits follows:

Time eaten _____

Food eaten _____

Were you hungry? Yes_____ No _____

Was this a "planned" food? Yes _____ No _____

Was this a highly processed food? Yes _____ No _____

Did this food satisfy you? Yes _____ No _____

What was your emotional feeling when eating? _____

The Harvard Health Publications website www.health.harvard .edu/staying-healthy/mindful-eating, can be a resource for further information on mindful eating.

Changing a Nutrition Lifestyle

Patients make changes when it is in their best interest to do so and it is up to the medical team to help each person recognize what is in their best interest. Food is the essence of life providing love, sense of belonging, economic status, and self-fulfillment. Many factors affect food choices but there is little study done on them because humans find it harder to study themselves than animals. Food science knows more about nutrient biochemistry than why people select specific foods, and more research focus has been on eating disorders of under-weight—anorexia nervosa or binge eating bulimia than obesity [3].

Bariatric surgery is meant to be an adjunct to a healthy diet and exercise regime. No single diet will please everyone but it needs to contain affordable nutrient-dense foods within their budget. Nutrient-dense foods are relatively expensive whereas high-calorie, low-nutrient foods are readily affordable. Habit changes are needed to encourage consumption of nutrient-dense foods despite the less-expensive, high-calorie products easily available. Food habits are ingrained early and unfortunately choices are determined by little more than a quick glance at the food label or mention of the product on television [4].

Regular Eating Habits

As David Ludwig, MD, PhD, in *Always Hungry?* states, "The science of nutrition seems to be stuck in the Dark Ages. While we've made many advances in the past few decades, in practice, very little has changed. We've discovered hormones that dramatically affect body weight. We've discovered sophisticated psychological theories about eating behavior. Machines can measure calories entering and leaving the body with precision. Yet we struggle to explain the ongoing obesity epidemic and suffer enormously from diet-related diseases"[5].

Dr. Ludwig's study in 1999 looking at high-glycemic foods and obesity should change everyone's idea of a healthy breakfast. He fed 12 young boys three different breakfasts of the same calorie level but with different carbohydrate levels. One breakfast was instant oatmeal (called a "whole grain" but a highly processed carbohydrate) versus steel-cut oats and the third breakfast of a vegetable omelet with fruit (no grain products and more protein and fat than the other two breakfasts). Blood glucose levels rose to very high levels from the instant oatmeal, a little less from the steel-cut oats and were low from the omelet and fruit breakfast [6].

In addition to the blood glucose response, Dr. Ludwig's research showed elevated adrenaline from the instant oatmeal breakfast, which caused hypoglycemic signs in the boys. The individuals who ate the instant oatmeal ended up eating significantly more at lunch when allowed to eat as much as they desired [6].

Similar studies [7–10] have shown the need for low-glycemic meals starting with breakfast to control appetite and cravings throughout the day. Limiting highly processed carbohydrates, especially at breakfast, is the best way to control hunger throughout the day.

Chowdhury et al. from the United Kingdom also emphasized the importance of breakfast in a study published in the *American Journal of Clinical Nutrition* [11]. Their study concluded that obese adults who ate a daily breakfast had greater physical activity during the morning whereas morning fasting resulted in dietary compensation later in the day. Insulin sensitivity increased with breakfast relative to fasting.

Eating Mindfully = Eating Slowly

Eating mindfully means eating slowly and paying attention to food textures, chewing, and swallowing, which is critical postbariatric surgery. Eating every 4–5 hours provides a stable energy level throughout the day and sets up a healthy appetite instead of ravenous hunger feelings at the sight of food.

Menu modifications are important when changing eating habits. Breakfast choices can include: homemade protein shake,* frittata or breakfast burrito, or homemade granola* with plain, full-fat yogurt. Lunch choices: chicken vegetable soup, salmon salad on rice crackers, or eggplant parmesan.* Dinner options: thyme roasted turkey and sweet potato, stir-fried chicken and vegetables, or fish with boiled potatoes and green beans. Desserts of fresh or cooked fruit (apples, peaches, or pears) topped with homemade granola.*

Cooking at Home

Americans spend more time and money eating outside the home than ever before. They spend about 50% of their food budget at restaurants now compared with 25% in 1955 according to the National Restaurant Association [12]. Eating at fast-food restaurants has been shown to be a major contributor to obesity, insulin resistance, and cardiovascular disease [13].

The excuse that many people give for increased meals away from home is that cooking is a challenging and time-consuming task they cannot fit into their busy lifestyles. Whether they lack the energy, time, or skills, the medical team needs to encourage more cooking at home through quick meal suggestions for better weight management and healthier food choices.

- Buy a good set of knives to cut and chop food.
- Prepare and cook big batches of food on weekends or time off so lunches and quick dinners are always available. (If it takes an hour to make four servings, then that is 15 minutes per meal that can fit into anyone's schedule.)
- Purchase fresh fruits and vegetables and wash them as needed instead of grabbing for chips, cookies, and snack bars.
- Plan for leftovers when preparing the evening meal.

Using Nutrition Labels

New food labels for food and beverages were proposed by food and drug administration (FDA) in the Federal Register March 3, 2014 but

---

* Since everyone likes recipes and menus at support meetings, the recipes are included in the Appendices.

deadlines for comments have been extended several times producing the agency's inability to publish a final rule for required label changes. Of particular interest is the proposed change on the label where added sugars are clearly displayed to allow consumers to identify calorie- and sugar-dense products. Serving sizes need modification because the current labels represent standards from the 1980s instead of consumption patterns today, especially when the full container is consumed [14].

The revised nutrition label will help bariatric surgery patients look at serving size, calories, fat content, and added sugars in a new way.

- Serving size will better reflect what a "normal serving" is instead of ice cream at 1/2 cup when a cup is a more usual amount than the consumer's scoop.
- Calories are noted in a bigger font on the label.
- Calories from fat have been deleted but the focus is on type of fat in the food since not all fats are created equal.
- Added sugars are listed directly on the label to provide a comparison of natural sugar versus added sweeteners.

Unfortunately, the food industry will use the "added sugar" listing on the nutrition panels to their advantage in confusing consumers about "natural" sweeteners. Consumers are recognizing sweeteners like stevia, monk fruit, and coconut sugar so these are going to be used as a replacement for sucrose. Blends of coconut sugar harvested from the coconut tree blossoms and water-extracted stevia called CoCoSweet is one of the new sweetener choices for food processors. Another stevia sweetener called EverSweet is being used in low-calorie products. Neither of these products are natural sweeteners. They are highly processed products obtained from fermentation methods used to entice consumers into eating and drinking foods that do not belong in a healthy diet [15].

Food and Socializing

Socializing and eating have been linked throughout the ages and pose big challenges for bariatric patients. They need to adapt a new habit of socializing **without** the need to eat whenever possible. Changing the social event to a nonfood format like a pool party or nature hike can be suggested by the patient to minimize food temptations. If a meal or snack is included, make it a healthy choice or suggest an alternative restaurant where nutritious choices are offered.

The process of living healthy applies to encouraging solitary dinner at a restaurant because *The Journal of Consumer Research* states we have more fun by ourselves when we get out of the house. Some bariatric patients feel they cannot socialize or eat out because of portion sizes, food choices, or dining alone. A growing segment of patients are single while others prefer to spend their eating time alone than with company.

Dining out successfully is an art for bariatric surgery patients. Here are several tips provided during support group meetings:

- Call ahead to the restaurant and have a menu sent to you so meal choices can be planned ahead
- Eat a healthy snack before going out to so you don't arrive hungry and only need to order soup or salad
- No bread basket on the table
- Select nonfried appetizer (shrimp cocktail), steamed spring rolls, or skewered chicken and vegetable kebob
- Be specific about how you want a meal item prepared
- Eat slowly and savor every bite
- Sip tomato juice while others eat rice and baked potato
- Share an appetizer and/or entrée

Changing Exercise Habits

The beverage giant Coca Cola advises everyone to not stress about cutting calories—just get more exercise. Yet study after study shows that exercise increases appetite and most people increase food intake to make up for whatever they exercised off.

Patients need to exercise for their health, not because it is good for weight loss. Coen and Goodpaster reviewed physical activity data for patients undergoing bariatric surgery and concluded that most of them do not exercise enough to reap the health benefits [16]. Exercise in Roux-en-Y gastric bypass (RYGB) surgery patients enhances mitochondrial respiration and improves insulin sensitivity [17].

Dikareva et al. explored the barriers that reduced physical activity among women who had undergone bariatric surgery. These barriers include mobility, side effects of surgery, body image problems, competing responsibilities, lack of exercise knowledge, and reduced access to facilities [18]. Zabatiero et al. also accessed bariatric surgery candidates and found most of them believed that physical activity provided health benefits but body pain, physical limitations, lack of motivation, and restricted resources provided barriers to participation in exercise [19].

On the other hand, exercise improves physical and mental health in bariatric surgery candidates according to Bond et al. using the health-related quality of life (HRQoL) survey [20]. Future studies need to access what can be done to improve compliance.

Sleep

According to a study in *SLEEP* about 40% of Americans are sleep deprived, meaning they get less than 5 hours of sleep per night. Maintaining a natural day and sleep cycle is fundamental for brain cells that synchronize the body clock. Skimping on sleep has long been associated with overeating, poor food choices, and weight gain. A recent study in *SLEEP* shows how this process changes chemical signaling in the blood and encourages eating sweet, salty, high-fat snack foods [21]. The study subjects were sleep-deprived and the endocannabinoid levels of the brain rose higher to enhance the desire for food.

Erin Hanlon, PhD, a research associate in endocrinology, diabetes, and metabolism at the University of Chicago points out that "the energy cost of staying awake a few extra hours seem to be modest." One study has reported that each hour of wakefulness uses about 17 extra calories. That adds up to about 70 cal for the 4 hours of lost sleep. But given the opportunity, the subjects in this study more than made up for it by binging on snacks, taking in more than 300 extra calories. Over time, that can cause significant weight gain [21].

Night shift workers have long been considered candidates for increased weight gain and chronic diseases. An estimated 15 million Americans work the night shift and the adverse health effects are well documented. Jonathan Cedernaes, MD, PhD, a researcher in the Department of Neuroscience at Uppsala University, Sweden indicates that shift workers showed signs of cognitive aging but this was not significantly different from nonshift workers. Dr. Cedernaes showed chronic sleep loss by shift workers can be repaid by choosing better quality sleep—avoiding caffeine, alcohol, and nicotine when catching up their sleep quota at other times [22].

Marie-Pierre St. Onge, PhD, assistant professor of medicine at Columbia University College of Physicians and Surgeons refutes the idea of sleep debt repayment. She asserts that short sleep duration on workdays is ubiquitous in today's society, so individuals try to catch up on sleep during weekends. Dr. St. Onge describes this behavior as "social jetlag"—the difference in sleep timing between workdays and free days. This behavior attempts to pay back over 2 days the deficit incurred during a 5-day work week, but studies have shown higher levels of obesity and metabolic syndrome due to increased body mass index (BMI) and fat mass, plus elevated C-reactive protein (a marker of inflammation) in the "social jetlag" group. [22].

The risk of diabetes increases with disruptions in a person's circadian rhythm reports Chandra L. Jackson, PhD, research associate with the Clinical and Translational Science Center at Harvard Catalyst and Harvard T.H. Chan School of Public Health. Type 2 diabetes risk was elevated for each hour of sleep lost among individuals who slept less than 7 hours per day. Dr. Jackson also reported that shift work where a person eats during the night is bad for metabolic health because the body releases hormones throughout the 24-hour period and glucose-insulin dysfunction may result when eating times differ from hormone releases. Weight gain and dysglycemia result [23].

Reduced weight loss in bariatric patients may be related to sleep deprivation because leptin and ghrelin issues are changing appetite and metabolism [24].

Leptin levels contribute to maintaining healthy appetite control but poor sleep contributes to poor leptin management. Ghrelin is the hunger hormone that is suppressed with sufficient sleep but increased during sleep deprivation.

Research over the past 15–20 years has begun to provide answers about why sleep is precious. Studies have explained that sleep provides optimal functioning of the immune system, hormonal balance, emotional, and psychological health, appetite regulation, memory, and learning plus clearance of toxins from the brain [25].

Obstructive sleep apnea (OSA) is a common disorder in obese patients who experience repetitive episodes of nocturnal breathing cessation due to upper airway collapse. Weight loss from bariatric surgery improves symptoms and can produce beneficial sleep [26].

Having good bedtime habits are important. Patients need to be advised to avoid eating late meals—allow at least 3 hours before bed. A light snack 30 minutes before bed is acceptable for those needing protein for blood glucose control. After dinner, mind and body activities need to avoid stimulating and agitative conversations including work stress to ensure better sleep. Small adjustments to the daily routine and sleeping area can go a long way to producing restful sleep and better health. A composite of suggestions include:

- Avoid television or computer-related activities at least 1 hour before bed.
- Sleep in a dark room.
- Use a low wattage yellow, orange, or red light bulb as a night light.
- Keep a cool bedroom temperature of 70°F–72°F.
- Take a hot bath before bed to increase core temperature and signal the body to sleep.

Sleep disorders often occur due to hormone imbalance or lack of physical activity. Stress and cortisol block the production of melatonin, which is needed to shift the brain from alpha wave sleep to deep delta waves. Supplements are available to help restore quality sleep. Magnesium also plays a role in sleep with low levels preventing the brain from quieting down for sleep. Zhou et al. report that consumption of a high-protein diet may improve sleep in overweight and obese adults [27].

Water Balance in the Body

Every cell in the body contains fluid and it is bathed in a sea of fluid resulting in the human body being 60%–65% water. These fluids are continually lost and need replacement because imbalances can be devastating to the metabolic system. Thirst is the primary response to influence water intake but dry mouth and signals from the hypothalamus may also trigger consumption [28].

When too much water is lost from the body and not replaced, dehydration develops causing weakness, exhaustion, and delirium or even death if not corrected [28]. The usual signs of dehydration are based on weight loss from fluids:

1%–2% fluid loss = thirst, fatigue, weakness

3%–4% fluid loss = impaired physical performance, dry mouth, reduced urine

5%–6% fluid loss = difficult concentration, headache, irritability, apathy, increased respiratory rate

7%–10% fluid loss = dizziness, spastic muscles, loss of balance, exhaustion, collapse

Water intoxification is rare but has been noted with excessive fluid ingestion. Symptoms of hyponatremia may occur in endurance athletes who incorrectly believe that overhydration can improve their stamina.

Water loss of about 500 mL (about 2 cups) per day as urine, feces, and perspiration is considered enough to carry away waste products from cell metabolism. Because fluid needs can vary based on diet, physical activity level, and environmental factors (temperature, humidity, altitude), a general water requirement is difficult to calculate. The usual recommendation is 2–3 L of water/fluid (7–11 cups) per day but it does not take into account dietary factors. The percentage of water in foods varies greatly so a processed food consumer will need more fluid than a salad lover.

Water in Selected Foods from USDA Database

- 90%–99%: Strawberries, watermelon, lettuce, cabbage, celery, spinach
- 80%–89%: Fruit juices, yogurt, apple, grapes, carrots
- 70%–79%: Shrimp, bananas, corn, potatoes, avocados, cottage cheese
- 60%–69%: Pasta, legumes, salmon, ice cream, chicken
- 50%–59%: Ground beef, hot dogs
- 40%–49%: Pizza
- 30%–39%: Bagel, bread, cheese
- 20%–29%: Cake, biscuits, crackers
- 10%–19%: Butter, margarine, dried fruit
- 1%–9%: Cereals, pretzels, peanut butter, nuts
- 0%: Vegetable oils

A study at the University of Illinois Urbana-Champaign campus, found that people who increased their consumption of water by one to three cups daily decreased their total energy intake by 68–205 cal daily while reducing sodium by 78–235 mg according to Recopeng An, PhD [29].

Stress and Anxiety

Researchers estimate that stress and anxiety have a lot to do with the inability to get a good night's rest. A study at the Johns Hopkins University School of Medicine, Baltimore found that people who awoke several times during the night had a worse mood in the morning than those who get the same amount of sleep without interruptions [30]. Mood and stress are challenges for those struggling with habit changes related to healthy eating and other lifestyle habits.

Stress may be the trigger in most instances of low mood, anxiety, and sleeplessness according to Vladimir Badmeav, MD, PhD, of American Medical Holdings. "The U.S. is the largest market for anxiety disorder therapeutics and supplements worldwide with the highest number of patients reporting anxiety disorders anywhere in the world" [31]. Dr. Badmeav noted that stress is one of the most significant health issues of the twenty-first century.

The human body produces cortisol as a stress response, which in turn results in anxiety, sleeplessness, low mood, and cognitive disruption. A typically busy lifestyle drains energy—mental and physical—which decreases quality of life and often times causes a sensation of feeling overwhelmed. The body's response to this metabolic stress can involve overeating, which sabotages the bariatric patient's success in losing weight.

Reducing stress by going for a walk instead of eating can have wide-ranging positive effects. Relaxation–response training can be taught during group sessions or private consultations through visualizations that aid weight management [32].

Principles for Better Health

Empowerment is the best investment that an individual needs to learn. The empowered bariatric surgery patient realizes they have the authority to manage their own health and the power to heal themselves through better habits. By becoming responsible for their own choices and creating a vision of themselves as healthy, they can proclaim these principles for a better quality of life in the future:

- Adequate sun exposure for Vitamin D
- Adequate and clean drinking water for hydration

- Eat REAL food (foods with labels are processed)
- Regular meal times—NOT 24/7
- Nourish mitochondria for energy and longevity
- Physical activity for bone and muscle
- Adequate sleep

Every bariatric surgery patient needs to keep motivated by

- Thinking wellness, not weight loss
- Setting realistic goals
- Dropping the "perfect" mentality
- Keeping a success journal

Ultimately, all patients know how to live healthy but these goals may be inconvenient and time consuming. Patients can dream up fool proof ways to override their new health decisions so support groups or a trusted health-care professional is the best way to help that individual tune out the noise of the food industry whose mantra is "Eat more, be happy." Such illusions lead to self-destruction and defeat. Self medication with food is a habit that needs to be changed in order to successfully monitor body weight.

CASE STUDY 1

AL is a 50-year-old male transit bus driver who reports he has already lost 20 lb. by changing his diet and watching what he eats. He has sleep apnea, hypertension, gastroesophageal reflux disease (GERD) and stress with his mother in a nursing home.

BMI: 41.1, body fat: 36.2 %, weight: 239.6 lb.

24-hour food recall of previous eating: Breakfast: donut; Lunch: skipped; Dinner: "making up for not eating lunch."

Current 24-hour food pattern: Breakfast: omelet, papaya, and pineapple cubes; Lunch: hard boiled eggs; Dinner: chicken and vegetables.

Nutrition counseling focused on complimenting him on excellent presurgery lifestyle changes. Provided additional menu tips and encouraged physical activity three times weekly.

CASE STUDY 2

GS is a 48-year-old male 4 years postadjustable gastric band-ing. He is a chef who describes himself as "having a passion for food." He takes warfarin but states he "eats anything he wants to" just not at fast-food restaurants.

BMI: 41.2, body fat: 32.8%, weight: 312.6 lb.

24-hour food intake: Breakfast: pastries, not eggs; Lunch: not identified; Dinner: "whatever appeals." He reports drinking a glass of wine daily and is resistant to reducing quantity.

His goal is "not wanting to be sick."

Nutrition counseling focused on regular eating plan with small high-protein food choices for RYGB surgery. He is famil-iar with 1–2 weeks of liquid diet based on gastric banding expe-rience but does not feel it is important to consume a liquid diet beyond the first week!

References

1. Farley TA. Fighting obesity is NOT just for kids. *New York Times Op-Ed.* Dec 18, 2015.
2. West DS, Di Lillo V, Bursac Z, et al. Motivational interviewing improves weight loss in women with Type 2 diabetes. *Diabetes Care* 2007;30:1081–1087.
3. Woldeyohannes HO, Soczynska JK, Maruschak NA, et al. Binge eating in adults with mood disorders: Results from the international mood disorders collaborative project. *Obes Res Clin Pract* 2015;24: S1871–403X(15)00161–1.
4. Wagner J. Why can't we all just eat healthy? *Nutritional Outlook.* July/August, 2009, p. 230.
5. Ludwig DS. Always hungry? Conquer cravings, retrain your fat cells and lose weight permanently. *Grand Central Publishing* 2016;16.
6. Ludwig DS, Majzoub JA, Al-Zahrani A, et al. High glycemic index foods, overeating, and obesity. *Pediatrics* 1999;103:E26.
7. Ludwig DS. Dietary glycemic index and obesity. *J Nutr* 2000;130:280s–283s.
8. Ludwig DS. Clinical update: The low glycemic-index diet. *Lancet* 2007;369:890–892.
9. Lennerz BS, Alsop DC, Holsen LM, et al. Effects of dietary glycemic index on brain regions related to reward and cravings in men. *AJCN* 2013;98:641–647.

10. Pawlak DB, Kushner JA, Ludwig DS, et al. Effects of dietary glycaemic index on adiposity, glucose homeostasis, and plasma lipids in animals. *Lancet* 2004;364:778–785.
11. Chowdhury EA, Ricardson JD, Holman GD, et al. The casual role of breakfast in energy balance and health: A randomized controlled trial in obese adults. *Am J Clin Nutr* 2016;103:747–756.
12. National Restaurant Association 2010. Restaurant Industry Pocket Factbook. Available at: www.restaurant.org.
13. Pueira MA, Kartashov AL, Ebberling CB, et al. Fast-food habits, weight gain and insulin resistance (the CARDIA study): 15 year prospective analysis. *Lancet* 2005;365:36–40.
14. Mermelstein NH. Gearing up for new nutrition labels. *Food Technology.* Jan, 2015;63–67.
15. Hartman L. Non-nutritive sweeteners see increased potential with new labels. *Food Processing.* Feb 18, 2016.
16. Coen PM, Goodpaster BH. A role for exercise after bariatric surgery? *Diabetes Obes Metab* 2016;18:16–23.
17. Coen PM, Menshikova EV, Distefano G, et al. Exercise and weight loss improve muscle mitochondrial respiration, lipid partitioning, and insulin sensitivity after gastric bypass surgery. *Diabetes* 2015; 64:3737–3750.
18. Dikareva A, Harvey WJ, Cicchillitti MA, et al. Exploring perceptions of barriers, facilitators, and motivators to physical activity among female bariatric patients: Implications for physical activity programming. *Am J Health Promot* 2015. [Epub ahead of print.]
19. Zabatiero J, Hill K, Gucciardi DF, et al. Beliefs, barriers and facilitators to physical activity in bariatric surgery candidates. *Obes Surg* 2016;26:1097–1109.
20. Bond DS, Thomas JG, King WC, et al. Exercise improves quality of life in Bariatric surgery candidates: Results from the Bari-Active trial. *Obesity* 2015;23:536–542.
21. Hanlon EC, Tasali E, Leproulth R et al. Sleep restriction enhances the daily rhythm of circulating levels of endocannabinoid 2-arachidonoylglycerol. *SLEEP* 2016;39930:653–664.
22. Cedernaes J. Can a sleep debt be repaid? *Endocrine Today.* Aug 13, 2015.
23. Jackson CL. Poor sleep habits as risk factor for diabetes, obesity cannot be ignored. *Endocrine Today.* Aug 12, 2015.
24. Taheri S, Lin L, Austin D, et al. Short sleep duration is associated with reduced leptin, elevated ghrelin and increased body mass index. In: Froguel P, ed. *PLOS Medicine* 2004;1:e62.
25. Stickgold R. Sleep on it. *Scientific American.* Oct 2015;313:52–57.
26. Spicuzza L, Caruso D, Di Maria G. Obstructive sleep apnoea syndrome and its management. *Ther Adv Chronic Dis* 2015;6:273–285.
27. Zhou Z, Kim JE, Armstrong CL, et al. Higher protein diets improve indexes of sleep in energy-restricted overweight and obese adults: Results from 2 randomized controlled trials. *Am J Clin Nutr* 2016;103:766–774.

28. Rolfes SR, Pinna K, Whitney E. *Understanding Normal and Clinical Nutrition*. Belmont, CA: Wadsworth, 2006, p. 396.

29. An R, McCaffrey J. Plain water consumption in relation to energy intake and diet quality among US adults, 2005-2012. J Human Nutr & Dietetics. Mar 2016.

30. Finan P. Bad Mood? Sleep Interruptions may be to blame. *Sleep*. Nov 4, 2015.

31. Schofield L. Addressing critical MASS (Mood, anxiety, stress and sleep). *Nutraceuticals World*. June 2015; 32–36.

32. Friedman R, Shackelford A, Reiff S, et al. Stress and weight maintenance: The disinhibition effect and the micromanagement of stress. In: Blackburn GL, Kanders BS, eds. *Obesity Pathophysiology and Treatment*. New York, NY: Chapman & Hall 1994, pp. 253–263.

13

FREQUENTLY ASKED QUESTIONS

Q: I have methylenetetrahydrofolate reductase (*MTHFR*) C677T and do not understand what Vitamin B_{12} and folate supplements I should take.

A: Vitamin B_{12} is also called cobalamin and the cheaper form is cyanocobalamin. Yes, it contains cyanide and it is found in most multivitamins but not in sufficient bioavailable quantity to improve mitochondrial function. A liquid or powder form of methylcobalamin B_{12} and methylfolate or 5-MTHFR is needed for MTHFR genetic single nucleotide polymorphisms (SNPs).

Q: The 2015 Dietary Guidelines for Americans recommendations are very different from the nutrition guidelines the nutritionist recommended after my bariatric surgery. What nutrition plan should I believe?

A: To quote David Katz, MD, Director of Yale University Prevention Research Center, "The *2015 Dietary Guidelines for Americans* are a national embarrassment. They are a betrayal of the diligent work of nutrition scientists, and willful sacrifice of public health on the altar of profit for well-organized special interests." The report focuses on food over nutrients but recommendations about what NOT to eat or limit is stated in terms of nutrients making it very confusing. Limiting the intake of saturated fat is prominently featured but with no indication of what foods to avoid or reduce. The same is true of added sugar. As Dr. Katz states, "Clearly advise about eating less of anything conflicts with the interests of some big industry sector of federal agencies and their bosses in Congress don't want to get upset. So somehow, we are left to cut back on our intake of saturated fat and sugar while washing down our corned beef with Coca-Cola."

Q: Do I need to be concerned about genetically modified organisms (GMO) foods?

A: The development and use of genetically engineered (GE) foods (also known as GMOs) is a controversial subject because long-term effects on humans are unknown and no federal law requires labeling food or ingredients if they are GMOs. Several major commodity crops are genetically altered: alfalfa, canola, corn, cotton, Hawaiian papaya or "solo" papaya, soy, sugar beets (used in granulated sugar), zucchini, and summer squash. GE apples and potatoes have been approved for sale but may not be available on the market yet.

A current estimate indicates that >90% corn, soy, and cotton acreage in the United States, is grown genetically engineered with products made from them used for infant formula, snack foods, ketchup, spaghetti sauce, and beverages made with high-fructose corn syrup, candy, and chocolate.

Genetic engineering has used billions of dollars for research and yet has not produced a healthier, more sustainable food supply, so who needs GMO food when research has shown weeds are becoming glyphosate-resistant (Round-Up)? Seeds are costlier because of patents, and seeds are artificially injected with foreign proteins that have never been tested.

Buy organic or GMO-free foods as often as possible since Americans are currently not allowed to know which foods contain modified genes. The Cauliflower Mosaic Virus (CaMV35s) promoter is used in most genetically engineered crops to activate foreign genes that have been inserted into the host. Just what we need is another virus in our metabolic system.

Q: Is obesity a disease?

A: Body weight is not a response to the law of physics but to the laws of biochemistry, so it is hard to classify it as a disease since it affects and contributes to many chronic disorders like cardiovascular disease, diabetes, hypertension, and cancer. During times in human history when food was scarce, our bodies developed the ability to store fat and weather the famine. Today, we have plenty of fat to burn, but society and technology has changed our eating and activity level. With lots more food available and less time needed to prepare it, weight gain abounds.

Q: A growing number of companies are offering wellness apps for employees to help them lose weight. Should I sign on?

A: Employers have been trying to get their employees to lose weight and eat better for a long time. The apps may offer a chance to help people individually make better choices instead of participating in a group session. But any kind of educational approach is only as effective as the motivation of the person participating. Dr. Jason Langheier, CEO and founder of Zipongo: Eating Well Made Simple, points out that the United States spends $8,500 per year for health care per person and $2000 on food and is ranked thirty-fifth globally for life expectancy. The Japanese spend $3,300 on health care and $3200 on food with a ranking of second in life expectancy.

Q: I do not know how to cook and have no time to learn how, so what do I do to help me lose weight after surgery?

A: Many Americans spend more time watching television than preparing their own meals. Studies show that those who prepare food at home have reduced incidence of obesity but they must dedicate the time and effort to cook a meal. If people can spend hours watching television, searching the Internet, and standing in line for the latest coffee creation, then they have the time to dedicate to their health and wellness by cooking nutritious meals at home along with getting some exercise.

Q: What is a healthy weight and waist circumference?

A: A healthy body mass index (BMI) is 18.5–25 kg/m² but anything less than 30 kg/m² is a desirable goal for bariatric surgery patients. Excess fat around the midsection or "belly fat" increases the risk for chronic diseases like cancer, stroke, heart disease, and diabetes. A waist circumference of 35 in. or less for women and 40 in. or less for men is desirable.

Q: What is the truth about fat?

A: Saturated fats are found in meats, cheese, and butter which are hard at room temperature. Eating large quantities of these foods can increase total blood cholesterol and low-density lipoprotein (LDL) cholesterol in some individuals. Coconut oil contains lauric acid, a medium chain triglyceride fat which lowers LDL cholesterol according to some research. *Trans* fats are a bad choice because they increase LDL and total cholesterol, and may reduce high-density lipoprotein (HDL) cholesterol. The hydrogenation of polyunsaturated fats like soybean and corn oil is what produces artificial *trans* fats and they need to be omitted from the diet.

Q: What about chocolate?

A: Dark chocolate contains stearic acid which is a saturated fat that does not raise LDL cholesterol, but it does not decrease it either. The *Journal of Nutrition* reported on health benefits of high-flavanol cocoa (the patent process cocoa from Mars identified by the flavanol symbol and statement on the package). Unfortunately, media reports about the "health benefits" of dark chocolate have failed to identify that not all dark chocolate contains healthy flavanols. The process of heating the cocoa powder destroys the flavanols and most chocolates are an unhealthy mixture of sugar and milk with a little cocoa powder stirred in.

Q: Why are processed foods not recommended?

A: Processed foods squander water, fertilizer, pesticides, seeds, fuel, and land resources needed to produce the ingredients in them. That is not sustainable and mindful eating. Mystery "meat" predominates in hot dogs, bologna, frozen dinners, and even veggie burgers. When profit is the motive in the food industry, quality ingredients are too expensive.

Q: How do I increase my Vitamin D?

A: Certain animal foods—fatty fish like salmon and mackerel and egg yolks—are good vitamin D sources. Sun exposure from May through September in the United States can help build your vitamin D levels. More than a billion people world-wide have insufficient or deficient vitamin D levels, including those who throw away the yolk of an egg and only eat the white. The American Heart Association is probably the biggest contributor to vitamin deficiency/insufficiency in the United States by limiting eggs and recommending only whites be consumed.

Individuals with darker skin pigmentation are at greater risk for Vitamin D insufficiency because the pigmentation slows the production in the skin. Low vitamin D levels have been associated with a higher risk of diabetes, heart disease, bone loss, and many cancers.

Q: My doctor told me to take calcium for my bones. What should I be taking?

A: Bones and teeth contain more than 90% of the body's calcium but this mineral is also important for muscle movement, nerve signaling, hormone activity, and blood flow. When the diet does not contain enough calcium from canned fish like sardines and salmon, yogurt can be a good source for those who can tolerate dairy products.

Many nondairy foods are fortified with calcium but the bioavailability has not been determined, especially in bariatric surgery patients.

Q: Everyone tells me physical activity is important if I want to lose weight and keep it off. I have never been active and don't know how to begin.

A: A support system is vital for success in starting a fitness or physical activity regime. Others serve as a support and cheering section especially as you look at low-intensity activities like walking or hiking to increase heart rate and help establish a habit of physical fitness.

Q: What can I do to treat my gastroesophageal reflux disease (GERD)?

A: Chronic heartburn or GERD can affect as many as 60%–70% of the obese population. Overeating increases the incidence of reflux disease as the stomach or the pouch is stretched and food stuffs get pushed into the throat.

GERD occurs when the sphincter muscle between that throat and the stomach allows stomach contents to reflux back up into the throat. The back-wash of acid, bile, and stomach contents irritates the lining of the throat and may lead to a condition called "Barrett's Esophagus."

The foods that can trigger GERD symptoms include alcoholic beverages, coffee, chocolate, peppermint, fried foods, spicy foods (chili, curry, salsa), and acid foods (tomato sauce, citrus fruits).

Q: A newspaper report stated that there is little evidence that beneficial bacteria from probiotics are safe and effective. Are probiotics a waste of money?

A: Probiotics have been getting bad press for years. Many health-care professionals do not realize how many studies have been done with probiotics and their effectiveness in irritable bowel syndrome (IBS) and *C. difficile* infection.

Sarah H. Yi, epidemiologist with the Centers for Disease Control and Prevention has been quoted as saying, "There's no research that definitely shows they are effective, certainly not enough to create guidelines for their use" in a recent *American Journal of Infection Control.* She obviously has not kept abreast of the numerous studies in *Pediatrics, Nutrition Metabolism, New England Journal of Medicine, American Journal of Clinical Nutrition*, and many other professional publications.

Q: Fasting has been recommended for quick weight loss while I await my bariatric surgery date. Is it safe to do?

A: David Ludwig MD, professor of nutrition at the Harvard T.H. Chan School of Public Health, says that a definite benefit of fasting is that it forces the body to shift from using glucose for fuel to using fat. The fat is then converted to ketones for energy that burns more efficiently than glucose. Long-term effects of fasting on weight loss have not been studied. Keep in mind that it takes a very disciplined person to skip meals everyday—whether those meals are breakfast, lunch, or dinner.

Q: Why do I have to eat whole fruit when drinking juice is easier?

A: Over the past 50 years, the concept of "juice" has changed from a beverage squeezed by hand to a commercial product that has been heated, pulverized, stored in large tanks, and reconstituted into "juice" before bottling. The concept of freshness has been replaced by a highly processed food devoid of the nutritional benefits found in whole fruits. Alissa Hamilton in her book *Squeezed: What You Don't Know About Orange Juice* reveals the shocking truth about the orange juice brands on the supermarket shelf. Cold pressed juices are more expensive and nutritious but whole fruit is your best choice.

Q: Why is alcohol restricted?

A: Gastroenterologist Bernd Schnabe and colleagues of the University of California San Diego School of Medicine found that chronic alcohol consumption suppresses a mouse antibacterial defense system in the intestine by blocking the ability to produce natural antibiotic proteins called regenerating islet-derived 3 beta (REG3B) and regenerating islet-derived 3 gamma (REG3G). According to their research, intestinal bacteria not only proliferate but migrate through the intestinal wall and can affect the liver. These mice had more severe liver disease as a result of the alcohol consumption. The study was reported in *Cell Host & Microbe* in February 10, 2016 issue.

Q: It feels like I am spending more and more on food with prices rising. Do I have to break the bank to provide nutritious food?

A: Plan your meals, use a shopping list, and skip convenience items to balance your food budget. If you prepare enough food for leftovers the next day, money can be saved. Shopping without a list leads to impulse buying instead of buying only what is needed. Convenience comes at a cost—about three times more expensive—so factor that in before buying. Skip the bags and tubs of pre-washed and cut produce and buy whole fruits and vegetables.

Organic foods cost more on average than conventional foods, so check out the Environmental Working Group's annual list of "dirty Dozen" fruits and vegetables that have the highest amount of pesticide residues.

Q: I buy only food that has "natural" on the label so that I know it is not processed and full of chemicals and GMO organisms. Is that the best guide?

A: People generally believe the word "natural" refers to food grown "in a natural way" like organic farming but nothing could be further from the truth. The use of "natural" on the food label is unregulated and food companies can use it to mean whatever they want. Kellogg's Kashi brand misled consumers with its natural claim for GoLean® Shakes that were composed of entirely synthetic and unnaturally processed ingredients according to a lawsuit filed on August 31, 2011. The Cornucopia Institute released a report "Cereal Crimes" in November 2011 detailing the presence of genetically engineered grains in a number of "natural" cereal brands, including Kellogg's Kashi. Purchasing organic is the safest and healthiest choice and, remember, the healthiest foods do not come with a label!

Q: What about the cellulose in grated cheese?

A: The addition of wood pulp cellulose to grated cheeses has been going on for **many** years but recently has gained consumer interest. Processed foods are not the safest and healthiest foods to select. Shaking a can of grated Parmesan cheese in a cardboard shaker to break up the lumps is made easier with cellulose but what about the economic fraud! Consumers believed they were buying a container of grated cheese—not a diluted cheese product containing wood pulp. Food And Drug Administration (FDA) even allows wood pulp from new trees to be called "organic." Check out chocolate syrup labels and most salad dressings. You will find cellulose as a thickener. Real food does not need a wood pulp thickener.

Q: Why is sleep so important?

A: Each day the brain, a small mass weighing only 3 lb., has to get rid of toxic protein wastes and debris as it gets ready for a new neurological challenge the next day. This waste disposal goes on nightly during sleep. If this plumbing system did not flush out waste products, protein clumps would form in the brain cells and lead to irreparable harm like Alzheimer's, Parkinson's, or other neurological diseases.

Sleep is just as important for the brain as for muscles. It is just that we know less about the astrocytes in the brain and spinal cord than we do about muscle cells. Jeffrey P. Barash, MD, medical director of the Valley Hospital Center for Sleep Medicine in Ridgewood, New Jersey warns that losing 2 hours of sleep is similar to the effect of alcohol intoxication, like difficulty in focusing, deterioration of work productivity, and impaired creativity.

APPENDIX I

KETOGENIC (LOW-CARBOHYDRATE) DIET

A ketogenic diet is a low-carbohydrate diet that offers many benefits including weight loss. The reduction of carbohydrates produces a metabolic state that increases efficiency for burning fat for energy. Ketones can also be used by the brain for energy. The ketogenic diet lowers blood glucose and improves insulin sensitivity without hunger.

Foods to avoid on a ketogenic diet include: sugar containing foods—soda, smoothies, cake, cookies, candy; grains and starches—rice, pasta, cereals, bread; beans and legumes—lentils, chickpeas, kidney beans; unhealthy fats—processed vegetable oils; alcohol; sugar-free and low-fat products—anything containing sugar alcohols and sugar substitutes.

Foods to eat include meat, chicken, turkey, fish, eggs, healthy fats (olive, coconut, avocado, butter), lots of vegetables, small amounts of fruit eaten with a protein.

A high-protein ketogenic diet helps bariatric surgery candidates lose weight and start focusing on protein foods as critical in their future meal planning.

Meal Planning for Ketogenic Diet

Protein: 8–10 oz. or 4 servings per day

- Egg = 1 oz.
- Fish, chicken, turkey, grass-fed beef, pork, lamb
- 2 slices well cooked bacon = 1 oz.
- Cheese 1 oz. per day

Vegetables: unlimited amount (except for starchy vegetables)

- Carrots, celery, broccoli, zucchini squash, lettuce, tomatoes, cucumbers
- Potato: 1 small

- Sweet potato: 1/2 small
- Winter squash and peas: 1/2 cup cooked

Fruit: 1–2 servings with meal

- No fruit juice or canned fruit
- 1/2 cup berries
- 1/2 grapefruit, 1 orange, 1 apple
- 12 grapes

Fats and oils: 3–6 servings (at least 1 at each meal for satiety)

- 1 tablespoon olive oil or avocado oil or nut oil = 1 serving
- 1/2 avocado = 1 serving
- 1 teaspoon mayonnaise = 1 serving

Dairy: 1/4–1/2 cup plain yogurt
Grains: NONE
Sweeteners: Stevia, monk fruit

Menu Ideas for Ketogenic Diet

Day 1 Breakfast: Bacon, eggs, 1/2 grapefruit
Lunch: Chicken salad with avocado on salad greens
Dinner: Baked salmon on steamed spinach with butter sauce, 1/2 cup mixed fresh berries
Day 2 Breakfast: Canadian bacon, 1/2 cup papaya cubes
Lunch: Tuna salad + olives on spring greens with sliced apple
Dinner: Baked chicken, 1/2 sweet potato + butter, green beans
or
Eggplant parmesan (see recipe) and salad
Day 3 Breakfast: Pork sausages + apple slices
Lunch: Shrimp cocktail + avocado cucumber salad and orange slices
Dinner: Flank steak, asparagus + tomato salad
Snacking choices: Guacamole and vegetables
Whole milk plain yogurt + 1/2 cup berries
Protein power shake (see recipe)

Protein Power Shake

2 tablespoons canned coconut milk
1/4 cup plain full fat yogurt
4 tablespoons whey protein powder
1/2 cup frozen berries—blueberries, raspberries, strawberries
1/2 ripe pear or banana or mango
1 tablespoon coconut oil or 1/4 ripe avocado
Puree all ingredients in blender until smooth. Serve immediately.
  Makes one serving.

Eggplant Parmesan

The ultimate Italian comfort food that can be made ahead, refrigerated, and cooked while reviewing the mail, or reheated as a quick lunch.

1 medium eggplant (about 1 lb.)
1 tablespoon extra virgin olive oil
12–16 oz. ground turkey, chicken, or beef
1 cup ricotta cheese
1 cup grated Mozzarella cheese
1 large zucchini squash, cut into 1/4-in.-thick slices
2 cups organic marinara sauce
2 tablespoons chopped fresh basil leaves
1/4 cup grated Parmesan cheese

  Cut eggplant into 1/4-in.-thick slices and coat with oil. Arrange on baking sheet. Roast in 350°F oven until tender, about 10–15 minutes. Saute ground turkey, cool and stir in ricotta and Mozzarella cheeses. Oil the bottom and sides of 9 × 13 in. baking pan. Layer 1/2 eggplant slices, 1/2 zucchini slices, and 1/2 meat and cheese mixture. Spread on 1 cup of marinara sauce with 1 tablespoon basil leaves. Repeat layering. Sprinkle Parmesan cheese on top and bake 25–30 minutes until bubbly. Makes four servings.

Appendix II
Mediterranean Diet and DASH Diet

The Mediterranean and dietary approaches to stop hypertension (DASH) diet are usually recommended to help individuals control lipids and blood pressure while learning to make healthier food choices. A Mediterranean diet emphasizes lean proteins (red meat usually limited to once a week), legumes, nuts, whole grains, and fruits and vegetables. The focus is on plant-based foods and the use of olive oil as a healthy fat. Bread is an important part of the diet—usually dipped in olive oil.

A Mediterranean diet typically includes a moderate amount of wine, usually red, but bariatric surgery patients are usually advised to limit or restrict alcohol use.

General menu guidelines include:

Protein: 4–6 oz. per day (one serving of fish/seafood at least 2 times/week)

- Chicken, turkey, grass-fed beef, pork lamb
- Salmon, tilapia, snapper, shrimp, lobster, clams, mussels
- 1 egg = 1 oz.
- 5 medium shrimp = 1 oz.
- Limit red meat to 1 serving/week or 1–2 times/month

Vegetables: 4–6 servings per day

- Broccoli, tomatoes, cabbage, carrots, green beans, salad greens
- 1/2 cup cooked = 1 serving
- 1 cup salad greens = 1 serving
- 1/2 cup raw vegetables = 1 serving

Fruit: 3 servings per day

- Orange, strawberries, apple, banana, blueberries, peach, papaya
- 1 piece fresh fruit = 1 serving

- 1/2 cup chopped fresh or frozen fruit = 1 serving
- 1/2 banana = 1 serving

Dairy: 1–2 servings per day (choose low fat)

- 1 cup milk or yogurt = 1 serving
- 1 oz. cheese = 1 serving

Whole grains: 3–4 servings per day

- 1 slice bread = 1 serving
- 1/2 cup rice or pasta = 1 serving
- 1/2 cup cooked oatmeal = 1 serving

Fats and oils and nuts: 3–4 servings

- Olive or nut oils 1 tablespoon = 1 serving
- Salad dressing 1 tablespoon = 1 serving
- 1/4 cup whole nuts = 1 serving

Menu Ideas

Day 1　Breakfast: Plain low fat yogurt + strawberries and homemade granola (see recipe)
Lunch: Cheese sandwich on whole grain bread + vegetables
Dinner: Eggplant cheese lasagna and fresh fruit

Day 2　Breakfast: Oatmeal with raisins or blueberries
Lunch: Tuna salad sandwich with olives and tomato
Dinner: Lamb chop, macaroni, and salad

Day 3　Breakfast: Omelet with vegetables + fresh fruit
Lunch: Salad with feta cheese and olives + fresh fruit cup
Dinner: Salmon, basmati rice, broccoli

Snacking choices　　Greek yogurt
Piece of fresh fruit
Apple slices with goat cheese

Homemade Granola

1 cup steel-cut oats
1/2 tablespoon sesame seeds
1/2 cup chopped nuts

1/4 cup unsweetened shredded coconut
3 tablespoons coconut oil or high oleic sunflower oil
1/2–1 teaspoon stevia sweetener

Combine oats, sesame seeds, nuts, and coconut in 9 × 13 in. baking pan. Combine oil and stevia in small bowl and drizzle over mixture. Stir to coat. Bake in 350°F oven 15–20 minutes or until golden brown. Stir as needed to brown evenly. Cool and store in air tight container until ready to eat. Makes 1½ cups.

Appendix III
Glycemic Index and Glycemic Load

The glycemic index (GI) and glycemic load (GL) is a means of qualifying the carbohydrates in the diet for treating a chronic disease called diabetes. Replacing high-glycemic foods with low-glycemic foods can have a significant influence on blood glucose levels and insulin responses that cause inflammatory processes in the body.

The GI is a method of identifying carbohydrate foods by their effect on glucose response. The GI ranks foods based on how they increase blood glucose levels 2–3 hours after eating. Carbohydrate foods are ranked 0–100 with low-glycemic foods containing carbohydrates slow to digest ranked less than 55, and high-glycemic foods 70 and above.

To determine a food's GI, a measured portion of food containing 50 g of carbohydrate is fed to 10 healthy people after an overnight fast. Fingerprick blood samples are taken at 15–30 minutes interval over the next 2 hours and the blood glucose response is calculated based on the average from all subjects per the University of Sydney, Australia, protocol. The International Tables of Glycemic Index was published by the *American Journal of Clinical Nutrition* in 1995 and 2002 followed by *Diabetes Care* in 2008.

A select listing of the GI of foods commonly consumed follows:

Breads	White	72
	Whole wheat	72
	Waffle	76
	Bagel	72

Cereals	Cheerios	74
	Cornflakes	83
	Oatmeal	49
	Oatmeal (1 min)	66
	Puffed rice	90
	Special K	54
Grains and pasta	Rice (instant)	91
	White rice	88
	Brown rice	82
	Sweet corn	55
	Rice cake	82
	Wheat Thins	67
	Rice pasta	92
	Macaroni	46
	Spaghetti	40
Desserts and sweets	Angel food	67
	Bran muffin	60
	Pound cake	54
	Honey	58
	Pretzels	83
	Popcorn	72
	Skittles	70
	Jelly beans	80
	Vanilla wafers	77
Dairy products	Ice cream	61
	Yogurt, plain	33
Fruit	Apple	38
	Banana	62
	Cantaloupe	65
	Grapefruit	25
	Orange	43
	Papaya	58
	Watermelon	72

Low-Glycemic Diet

A low-glycemic diet is frequently used for individuals with prediabetes or type 2 diabetes and those with elevated triglycerides. Carbohydrate food choices should have a low GI from the listing above.

Protein: 8–10 oz. or 4 servings per day (including egg and dairy)

- Natural cheeses
- Plain yogurt: 8 oz = 1 serving
- Fish, chicken, grass-fed beef, lamb, pork
- Egg: 1 = 1 oz.

Fruit: 2 fresh or 2 ½ cup servings frozen (NO canned fruit)

- Low-GI choices: apple, orange, grapefruit, tangerine (limit high-glycemic choices to small amounts—banana, watermelon)
- No fruit juices or dried fruit
- Consume fruit with meal to reduce glycemic effect

Nonstarchy vegetables: Unlimited amounts

- Carrots, celery, broccoli, zucchini squash, lettuce, cucumbers, radishes

Starchy vegetables and grain-based foods: 2–3 servings per day

- Cooked whole grains: 1/2 cup brown rice, wild rice, basmati rice, millet, quinoa, rolled oats
- 1/2 cup serving sweet potato/yam, winter squash, turnip, pumpkin
- 4 whole grain crackers = 1 serving
- 1 slice bread = 1 serving

Healthy fats: 3–5 servings per day

- Olive oil, nut oils : 1 tablespoon = serving
- Avocado
- Nuts and nut butters: 5 almonds = 1 serving or 1 tablespoon almond butter
- 5 olives = 1 serving

Sugary beverages, candy, alcohol: NONE

Menu Ideas for Low-Glycemic Diet

Breakfast   1/2 cup cooked steel-cut oats with 1/2 cup berries
Lunch   Chicken salad with 4 whole grain crackers
              Spring greens and tomato salad with olive oil dressing
              Apple
Dinner   Broiled fish with lemon
              Basmati rice with toasted pine nuts
              Steamed broccoli
Snack   Popcorn

Glycemic Load

The GL concept is used to describe how combinations of foods can affect blood glucose response. A low-GL diet contains nonstarchy vegetables and legumes as key carbohydrate sources. A moderate-GL diet contains fruits, dairy products, and unsweetened breads and cereals. The high-GL diet has sweetened cereals, doughnuts, pancakes with syrup, candy, cookies, and sweetened beverages.

The GI assists in better food selection and the GL aids in development of healthy meal planning. Modifying carbohydrate foods in the diet can influence weight loss in addition to blood glucose response. Low-GL meals of low-GI foods can optimize hormones that regulate appetite.

The protein power shake and homemade granola recipes are good examples to offer bariatric surgery candidates during support group meetings.

APPENDIX IV
Low FODMAP Diet

The low-fermentable oligo-, di-, and monosaccharides, and polyols (FODMAP) diet is gaining acceptance for treating gastrointestinal disorders that may be a factor in candidates pre- and post bariatric surgery. Ingesting foods with these carbohydrates is believed to cause gastrointestinal symptoms like gas, bloating, pain, and irregular bowel movements, commonly called irritable bowel syndrome (IBS) and inflammatory bowel disease (IBD).

Use of a diet limited or restricted in long chain carbohydrates from sugar, cereal grains, legumes, and cruciferous vegetables (Brussels sprouts, cabbage, kale, broccoli) began over 50 years ago as a possible treatment for celiac disease and was made popular by various authors including Elaine Gottschall. Four specific carbohydrate types: (1) oligosaccharides, (2) disaccharides, (3) monosaccharides, and (4) polyols are poorly absorbed in the intestinal tract, which facilitates the overgrowth of bacteria and yeast. Consequently, excess mucus secretion and inflammation damage the intestinal lining and cause symptoms.

Oligosaccharides include fructose and galactose, which are commonly found in wheat, rye, onions, legumes, and cruciferous vegetables. Prebiotic nutrition supplements also contain oligofructans and may cause symptoms in bariatric surgery patients who are using probiotics with added prebiotics.

Disaccharides are two-linked sugars primarily found in dairy products containing lactose. Without adequate lactase enzyme, lactose intolerance causes discomforting gastrointestinal symptoms.

Monosaccharides are the simplest form of carbohydrate—glucose, fructose, galactose. Fructose is the most problematic dietary monosaccharide with about half of the U.S. population exhibiting malabsorption when 25 g or more are consumed according to Gibson PR et al. in *Alimentary Pharmacology Therapy* (2007) [1].

Many protein nutrition products used pre- and post bariatric surgery contain significant levels of FODMAPS, which can produce intestinal problems like diarrhea, bloating, and abdominal pain.

The FODMAPs in the diet are predominately found in

- Fructose—fruits, honey, high-fructose corn syrup
- Lactose—dairy products
- Fructans—wheat, garlic, onion, inulin
- Galactans—legumes (beans, lentils, soybeans, chick peas)
- Polyols—sweeteners (isomalt, mannitol, sorbitol, xylitol, avocado, apricots, cherries, nectarines, peaches, plums)

FODMAPs are osmotic so they pull water into the intestinal tract during digestion; however, many of them are not digested but are fermented by bacteria. When consumed in high amounts, gastrointestinal distress results in diarrhea, gas, or cramping and can even lead to constipation.

High FODMAPs Foods

- High-fructose corn syrup (HFCS)
- Dairy: buttermilk, chocolate milk, ice cream, milk, soft cheese (cottage, ricotta), sour cream
- Nuts: cashews, pistachios
- Legumes: lentils, beans
- Grains: wheat, barley, rye, spelt
- Fruits: apples, apricots, blackberries, dates, canned fruit, dried fruit, figs, mango, papaya, peaches, pears, plum, prunes, watermelon
- Vegetables: artichoke, cauliflower, mushrooms, peas
- Beverages: soda with HFCS, wine coolers, sherry, port

Low FODMAPs Foods

- Eggs, meat, chicken, shellfish, fish, lamb
- Dairy: cream cheese, hard cheeses (cheddar, parmesan), mozzarella, yogurt
- Nuts: macadamia, walnut, pecans, pine, coconut

- Grains: oatmeal, popcorn, quinoa, rice
- Fruits: bananas, blueberries, cantaloupe, cranberries, grapes, honeydew, kiwi, lemon, orange, pineapple, raspberries, rhubarb, strawberries, tangerine
- Vegetables: bell peppers, carrots, green beans, kale, cucumbers, cabbage, lettuce, parsnips, potatoes, radishes, seaweed, spinach, squash, tomatoes, turnips, zucchini
- Coffee, tea

Low FODMAPs Menu Guide

Day 1   Breakfast: Poached egg on spinach, gluten-free toast
        Lunch: Sliced turkey on gluten-free bread, sliced tomato and tangerine
        Dinner: Baked fish, rice, carrots, papaya slice, salad
Day 2   Breakfast: Corn flakes and banana with coconut milk
        Lunch: Frittata and salad
        Dinner: Baked chicken, sweet potato, green beans, blueberries
Day 3   Breakfast: Gluten-free waffle with fresh berries and bacon
        Lunch: Gluten-free pizza with mozzarella cheese
        Dinner: Lamb chop, baked potato, squash medley, salad
Snacking choices: Rice cakes with cream cheese
                    Banana
                    Grapes

Reference

1. Barrett JS, Irving PM, Gibson PR et al. Comparison of the prevalence of fructose and lactose malabsorption across intestinal disorders. *Aliment Pharm Ther* 2009; 30(2): 165–1174.

Index